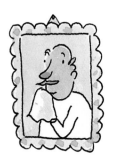

HEALTH AND HEALING
THE NATURAL WAY

---

# FIGHTING
# ALLERGIES

---

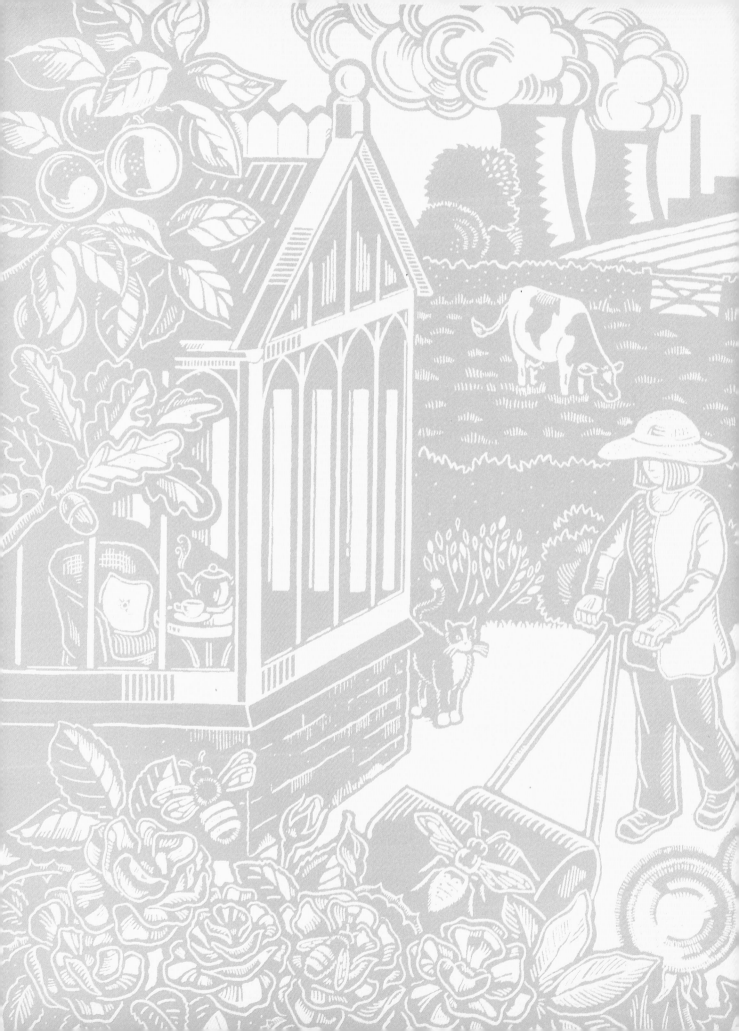

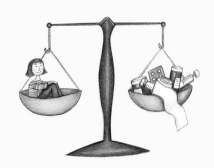

## HEALTH AND HEALING
## THE NATURAL WAY

# FIGHTING ALLERGIES

PUBLISHED BY

THE READER'S DIGEST ASSOCIATION, INC.

PLEASANTVILLE, NEW YORK / MONTREAL

## A READER'S DIGEST BOOK
Produced by
Carroll & Brown Limited, London

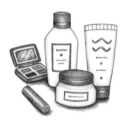

### CARROLL & BROWN

**Publishing Director** Denis Kennedy
**Art Director** Chrissie Lloyd
**Managing Editor** Sandra Rigby
**Managing Art Editor** Tracy Timson
**Editor** Joel Levy
**Art Editor** Simon Daley
**Designer** Evie Loizides
**Photographers** David Murray, Jules Selmes
**Production** Wendy Rogers, Clair Reynolds
**Computer Management** John Clifford, Karen Kloot

Printed in the United States of America

Library of Congress Cataloging in Publication Data

Fighting allergies.
        p.  cm. — (Health and healing the natural way)
    Includes index.
    ISBN 0-7621-0264-0
    1. Allergy—Treatment. 2. Allergy—Alternative treatment.
3. Allergy—Homeopathic treatment.
I. Reader's Digest Association.    II. Series.

RC584.F49 2000
616.97'06—dc21                              99-047859

Address any comments about *Fighting Allergies* to
Editor in Chief, U.S. Illustrated Reference Books,
Pleasantville, NY 10570.

The information in this book is for reference only;
it is not intended as a substitute for a doctor's diagnosis and care.
The editors urge anyone with continuing medical problems
or symptoms to consult a doctor.

### CONSULTANTS

Dr. Honor M. Anthony MB ChB
*Specialist in Environmental Medicine, Leeds*

Roger Newman Turner BAc, ND, DO
*Member of the Register of Naturopaths*
*Member of the Register of Osteopaths*

### CONTRIBUTORS

Dr. Paul J. August FRCP *Consultant Dermatologist*

Dr. Keith K. Eaton LRCPE, LRCSE, LRFPSG
*Consultant Allergist, Princess Margaret Hospital, Windsor*

Dr. David L.J. Freed MB, ChB, MD, CBiol, MIBiol
*Consulting Allergist, Salford Allergy Clinic*

Dr. D. Jonathan Maberly FRCP, FRACP
*Consultant Physician*
*Medical Director of the Airedale Allergy Centre*

Dr. John R. Mansfield LRCP, MRCS, DRCOG
*Consultant Allergist, Burghwood Clinic*

Dr. Michael J. Radcliffe MB, ChB, MRCGP, FAAEM
*Associate Specialist in Allergy, Middlesex Hospital*

Dr. Michael A. Tettenborn MB, FRCP, FRCPCH
*Consultant in Paediatrics and Child Health,*
*North Downs NHS Trust*

Dr. Richard Turner MB, MRCP
*Specialist in Allergy, North Hampshire Hospital, Basingstoke*

### READER'S DIGEST PROJECT STAFF

**Series Editor** Gayla Visalli
**Editorial Director, health & medicine** Wayne Kalyn
**Design Director** Barbara Rietschel
**Production Technology Manager** Douglas A. Croll
**Editorial Manager** Christine R. Guido
**Art Production Coordinator** Jennifer R. Tokarski

### READER'S DIGEST ILLUSTRATED REFERENCE BOOKS, U.S.

**Editor-in-Chief** Christopher Cavanaugh
**Art Director** Joan Mazzeo
**Operations Manager** William J. Cassidy

### READER'S DIGEST BOOKS & HOME ENTERTAINMENT, CANADA

**Vice President and Editorial Director** Deirdre Gilbert
**Managing Editor** Philomena Rutherford
**Art Director** John McGuffie

# Fighting Allergies

**M**ore and more people today are choosing to take greater responsibility for their own health care rather than relying on a doctor to step in with a cure when something goes wrong. We now recognize that we can influence our health by making improvements in lifestyle, for example, improving our diet, getting more exercise, and reducing stress. People are also becoming increasingly aware that there are other healing methods—some of them new, others ancient—that can help prevent illness or be used as a complement to orthodox medicine.

The series *Health and Healing the Natural Way* will help you to make your own health choices by giving you clear, comprehensive, straightforward, and encouraging information and advice about methods of improving your health. The series explains the many different natural therapies that are now available, including aromatherapy, herbalism, acupressure, and a number of others, and the circumstances in which they may be of benefit when used in conjunction with conventional medicine.

*Fighting Allergies* surveys the complex and often controversial subject of allergies. Some of the medical practitioners and researchers working in this field regard allergies as the next major health issue in the developed world, but for many of the millions suffering today the available diagnostic methods may be inadequate. *Fighting Allergies* presents both conventional and complementary therapies used for the management of allergies and also surveys the lifestyle, environmental, and dietary issues that underlie many problems of allergy. It aims to provide the information you need to understand allergies, and explains how to detect and manage allergic conditions. More than this, it reveals the range of both everyday and serious illnesses that may be caused, either partly or entirely, by allergy and highlights the complex interactions between diet, environment, and lifestyle in general health.

# CONTENTS

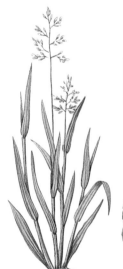

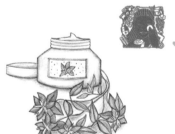

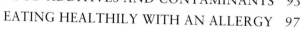

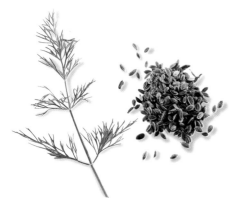

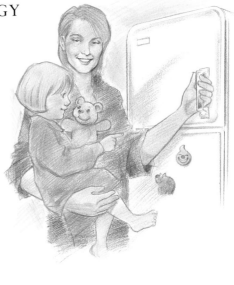

# ALLERGY ALERT

*Evidence suggests that allergies may become the major health issue of the 21st century. There are steps you can you take to protect yourself and your family.*

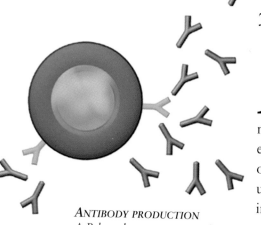

**ANTIBODY PRODUCTION**
*A B-lymphocyte—a type of immune cell—acts as an antibody-producing factory, making the antibodies that can be the key players in allergic reactions.*

**EDWARD JENNER (1749–1823)**
*In 1796 this English physician developed the technique of vaccination against smallpox. Public demonstrations, like the one shown below, helped to convince the medical establishment of the value of his work.*

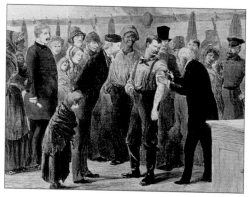

Allergies are often perceived as little more than a minor irritation. But it is becoming increasingly apparent that well-known conditions, such as hay fever and asthma, may be just the tip of an allergy iceberg. There is now considerable evidence that allergies could be causing or exacerbating a wide range of physical and mental disorders, but as yet this possibility remains unrecognized by many orthodox physicians. How can such an important health issue be so marginalized? The roots of the controversy stretch far back into medical history.

In 1906 a Viennese physician named Clemens von Pirquet coined the term "allergy" to describe the adverse immune reaction (serum sickness) that repeatedly vaccinated children developed to a substance that should have been harmless. Similar adverse reactions had previously been noted by the Romans, ancient Greeks, and medieval Chinese, but von Pirquet put a name to the condition. What lay behind his discovery?

## THE HISTORY OF ALLERGIES

In medieval times some physicians observed that if a person recovered from the plague, he or she would subsequently be immune to it. During the same period in China a crude form of immunization for smallpox, called variolation, was developed. The technique was introduced to Europe in the 18th century, but carried considerable risks and was soon supplanted by vaccination, a method developed by the English doctor Edward Jenner.

It was not until the 19th and 20th centuries that scientific discoveries helped to uncover how this new technique was capable of conferring immunity to disease. It was found that the state of immunity was due, at least in part, to protein molecules in the blood called antibodies, and that the production of antibodies is caused by the presence of a foreign body, or antigen—

normally a harmful substance, such as a virus or bacterium. However, it was also found that nondangerous, noninfectious materials, like pollen or even foods, could give rise to antibody formation. Injecting a serum that contained antibodies could be life-saving, but if a patient needed several injections of that serum over a few days or weeks, the result was the painful and sometimes life-threatening serum sickness. Von Pirquet noticed this effect, and thus gave us the term "allergy" to describe it.

Before long it became clear that skin rashes that appeared on some people after eating strawberries or shellfish and sneezing attacks caused by exposure to pollen also resulted from this changed reactivity, and doctors realized that these conditions were also the result of an allergic reaction.

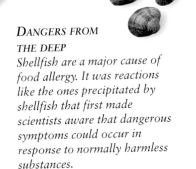

**DANGERS FROM THE DEEP**
*Shellfish are a major cause of food allergy. It was reactions like the ones precipitated by shellfish that first made scientists aware that dangerous symptoms could occur in response to normally harmless substances.*

## THE ROOTS OF CONTROVERSY

Once allergies had been recognized, scientists went to work on identifying the elements of the immune system that are involved and the mechanisms that underlie allergic reactions. By the late 1960s the antibody responsible for such classic allergic reactions as hay fever and skin rashes had been identified and named immunoglobulin E (IgE). This discovery marked the movement of the discipline into an increasingly strict scientific mode, with demarcations between what is considered an allergy and what is not.

As the scientific approach to allergies became more rigid, some doctors became increasingly aware that their clinical experience was at odds with conventional dogma. At the forefront of this group was Dr. Theron G. Randolph, an American physician whose clinical observations led him to believe that at least 30 percent of his patients were suffering from allergies. By paying careful attention to their diets and their working and living environments, he was able to identify trigger substances that conventional allergists did not recognize, and, by reducing his patients' exposure to them, he managed to cure illnesses that conventional medicine did not even recognize as allergic disorders. Randolph founded the discipline of clinical ecology (known as environmental medicine in

**DISCOVERERS OF IgE**
*In 1967 Teruko and Kimishige Ishizaka identified gamma E globulin, an antibody responsible for hay fever, eczema, and asthma, which later became known as IgE. This discovery provided the basis for scientific support for the study of allergies.*

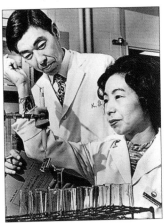

the United Kingdom), and was immediately marginalized by a suspicious medical establishment. Despite this reaction, the environmental hypothesis, as it is known in some circles, has continued to gain strength as the incidence of all kinds of allergies, or sensitivities, has skyrocketed.

## THE SCALE OF THE PROBLEM

While environmental allergists agree with conventional allergists on the theory of what constitutes an allergy, they disagree over how the available evidence fits into that theory. As a result, medical practitioners who focus on the environment are more open-minded about what can cause allergies and the conditions that may result from them.

What is not in dispute by either side is that the scale of the problem is growing and that allergies now affect large numbers of the world's population. In London 46 percent of adults tested had a positive allergy skin test in 1988, twice as many as in 1974, a doubling in only 14 years. In North America nearly 60 million people presently have asthma or other allergy-related conditions.

Figures for hidden, or delayed, food allergies and chemical sensitivities are hard to come by because few governmental health institutions recognize them as clinically authenticated conditions. But the data for what might be termed "classical allergies"—conditions like hay fever and asthma—tell the story just as clearly. The first case of hay fever was described in medical literature in the early 1800s, and the disease has since become increasingly common. In North America there has been an increase in rhinitis over the past 20 years, to the point where it now affects 10 to 13 percent of the population. Clinical experience suggests that there have also been increases in other chronic disorders that are allergy related. What lies behind these extraordinary figures?

## THE ENVIRONMENTAL HYPOTHESIS

Although the increase in chronic illnesses started in the West, it is now spreading to Third World countries as they become more developed. Could elements of the modern lifestyle be responsible? Environmental allergists offer several hypotheses that relate to our diet and environment and how we are changing them.

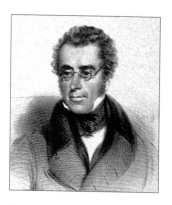

**JOHN BOSTOCK**
*In the summer of 1819 John Bostock spoke to the Royal Medical Society of London about his "periodical affection of the eyes and chest," which he referred to as "summer catarrh." The condition later became known as hay fever.*

**A DEVELOPING PROBLEM**
*Lifestyles in the developed world may be at the root of an increase in allergies. In South Africa hay fever is unknown among Xhosa tribespeople, like these women, who remain in their homelands. When they migrate to cities, however, great numbers of their children develop hay fever.*

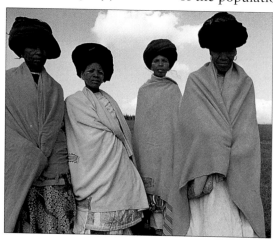

Perhaps the most wide-ranging change has been the makeup of our diets. Some allergists believe that we evolved over hundreds of thousands of years to eat only what we could hunt or gather—in other words, the diet consumed by our Stone-Age ancestors. Since the introduction of agriculture—and more recently, modern storage methods and rapid worldwide transportation—the elements of our diet have changed to include many foods that were not available in the past, or were available only rarely, and that the human body is therefore possibly ill-equipped to deal with. These include milk, eggs, potatoes, and cereals, not to mention preservatives and additives. This theory could explain why these items top the lists of trigger foods (see Chapter 4).

Human activities are causing the buildup of several different types of contamination, including outdoor pollution from industrial and traffic fumes; indoor pollution from cigarette smoke, synthetic fabrics and carpets, pets, molds, and dust mites; food and water contamination from pesticides, fertilizers, and additives; and pharmaceuticals, such as medications, perfumes, and makeup. In addition to drastically increasing the level of potential chemical triggers to which we are exposed, such pollutants could be changing the nature of our immune systems and making us more susceptible to allergies (see Chapter 3).

**CAVEMAN CUISINE**
*Fish, meat, and certain fruits, tubers, and herbs are believed to have been the main foods our Stone Age forebears would have eaten and thus the foods that our digestion systems are evolutionarily equipped to deal with.*

## WHAT DO DIFFERENT THERAPIES HAVE TO OFFER?

Although there are many conventional drugs and medications available for the treatment of disorders like hay fever, asthma, and eczema, many patients find that these drugs provide only temporary relief, need to be taken in increasing doses (with increasingly serious side effects), and can sometimes cause problems themselves. In addition, many doctors do not recognize chronic ailments as allergies and depend on medication to suppress the symptoms without treating the underlying causes.

For many people, complementary treatments for allergies, of which there are a number, offer a gentler and more natural alternative to conventional medications. Herbal remedies can be used to treat internal disorders, as well as to soothe skin problems like rashes. Aromatherapy, yoga,

**STEAM RELIEF**
*A face sauna clears the sinuses and helps to wash away irritating pollen. Natural remedies like this can provide alternatives to drugs in the management of rhinitis and other allergic conditions.*

acupuncture, and relaxation techniques may help directly with symptoms and can also play an important role in reducing stress. As helpful as all these therapies can be, however, they are limited to alleviating symptoms, without getting to the root of a problem.

## WHAT CAN YOU DO?

There is a whole range of strategies that can help you cope with and manage allergies and reduce the risk of developing any in the first place. You can learn to recognize the threat of allergy, find out where to seek help, and identify potential triggers and how best to avoid them. *FIGHTING ALLERGIES* provides the information you need to help you achieve these goals. The emphasis of the book is on practical steps you can take and on the therapies—both conventional and complementary—that you can use to treat and alleviate symptoms.

*T'AI CHI*
*The relaxing and energy-boosting benefits of t'ai chi, an ancient martial art, have been proven to help relieve a number of conditions, including asthma.*

Chapter 1 provides an explanation of the biology of allergies and a guide to the various methods used to test for and diagnose them.

Chapter 2 gives an overview of the strategies available for treating allergies, both conventional and alternative.

The next five chapters deal with the different groups of allergens that you might encounter and the disorders related to them.

Chapter 3 covers airborne allergens, from dust mites and pollen to chemicals and fumes. It also includes the two major allergic disorders of respiration—hay fever and asthma. Chapter 4 discusses the controversial subject of food allergy, and explains how diet has the potential to cause or cure a whole range of problems. Chapter 5 looks at allergic reactions of the skin, with particular focus on the substances that we come in contact with and the general problems of eczema, dermatitis, and urticaria. Chapter 6 considers drug allergies and how to reduce the need for medication to avoid the attendant problems. Chapter 7 contains a round-up of other sources of allergic triggers, including insects, and focuses on the deadliest of all allergic reactions, anaphylactic shock, also known as anaphylaxis. Chapter 8 looks at the special problems of children and allergies, in particular the issue of hyperactivity and related disorders.

Chapter 9 offers a directory of allergic disorders. This is a ready reference guide to help you find the information you need about an illness, how allergies might be involved, and how to prevent and treat allergic health problems.

# ARE YOU INFORMED ABOUT ALLERGIES?

*Allergy is a complicated subject, about which many people, including some doctors, are underinformed. For anyone who suffers from chronic illnesses and debilitating attacks, this lack of knowledge can be very serious. Learning about allergies could be the most important step you take to safeguard your health.*

Q **DO YOU HAVE CONSTANT, UNEXPLAINED SYMPTOMS?**
If you feel ill much of the time but your symptoms are vague and tend to come and go, and if your doctor has not been able to diagnose the problem, you might do well to consider the possibility of allergies. Many allergy patients have bulging medical files filled with notes on past ailments that did not seem to have any physical cause. Their symptoms might include fatigue; unexplained fevers, aches, and pains; mood swings; rashes that come and go; unexplained itching; and intermittent digestive upsets. Yet a doctor can never find much wrong. Some doctors label such patients as difficult or dismiss their symptoms as psychosomatic. Chapter 2 tells you where to seek help to find out if you have an allergy, and Chapter 9 explains why some doctors are reluctant to entertain the notion that allergies could be causing diverse but seemingly unrelated symptoms.

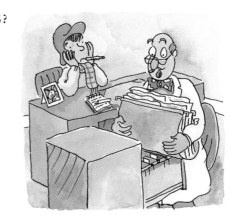

Q **SHOULD YOU BE WORRIED ABOUT ALLERGIES?**
Media interest in individuals who have multiple allergies (see Chapter 7) may alarm people who suspect that they, too, might be allergic to many things. Issues such as what you can safely eat may also be worrying, but before attributing your symptoms to allergy, you need to look at the evidence. Although there are many clues that indicate allergy, few are conclusive. The sort of vague and wide-ranging symptoms described above might strongly suggest an allergy. Chapters 3 to 7 describe possible allergic symptoms in detail. The markers that parents should look for when considering whether their children could have allergies are outlined in Chapter 8. Professionals can call on a range of tests to help them diagnose allergies, from prick and patch tests to alternative techniques like kinesiology (see Chapter 1). The best route to diagnosis is to conduct double-blind trials of foods and chemicals, possibly following special diets that eliminate typical allergenic foods (see Chapters 1 and 4).

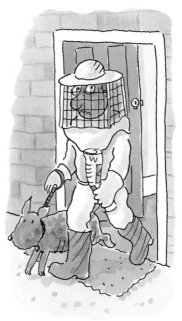

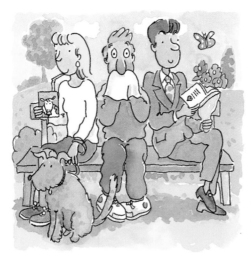

## Q WHY DO SOME PEOPLE HAVE ALLERGIES AND OTHERS DO NOT?

Even experts cannot fully explain why some people have allergies, while others are free of them; the issue is complicated. Genetics definitely plays some part, but exactly how large a part is not clear (see Chapter 1). Exposure to potential triggers in the first years of life—including the time in the womb—seems to be important. This means that what your mother ate, drank, and came into contact with could have been vital in determining your present allergic status (see Chapters 1 and 8). Frequency of contact with allergens is also significant; the most common allergens tend to be the ones that are found everywhere (see Chapters 3 to 6).

## Q WHAT IF MY DOCTOR DOESN'T BELIEVE IN FOOD ALLERGY?

All physicians recognize immediate food reactions, such as the anaphylactic shock that some people experience after eating peanuts. But delayed reactions, in which foods cause symptoms not normally associated with the gut—arthritis, mood swings, or fluid retention, for example—after several hours, or even days, are a different matter. Despite a wealth of evidence to the contrary, many doctors dismiss the idea that foods can produce such reactions. Even doctors sympathetic to the idea of food allergy may consider only a limited range of potential triggers. You may have to raise the issue yourself, in which case, you will need to learn as much as possible about food allergies. You may even have to find out where to obtain alternative professional support. Chapter 4 gives detailed information on where to find help for a food allergy.

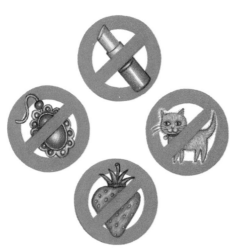

## Q WHAT CAN I DO TO EASE MY SYMPTOMS?

Once you have determined which substances trigger your allergic reactions, the first step should be to minimize your contact with them. In some instances this can be quite simple; for example, if you are allergic to a certain makeup, you can simply stop using the product. Other allergies, such as those involving certain foods, can be more disruptive; they require special diets and the need to shop and cook with the allergy in mind (see Chapter 4). Perhaps the most difficult allergies to cope with are those involving the environment, such as reactions to pollens or chemicals in the air. Avoiding pollen, dust mites, chemicals, and pet dander can be difficult, but even in these cases there are precautions you can take and treatments that will help provide relief from symptoms (see Chapter 3).

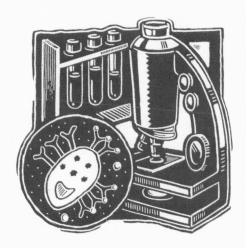

# CHAPTER 1

# EXPLAINING ALLERGIES

*Ever since allergies were first recognized in the early part of the 20th century, they have attracted controversy. What constitutes an allergy, which substances can cause one, and how should a sufferer be treated? This chapter presents the basic knowledge you will need to understand what different people mean by the term "allergy."*

# WHAT IS AN ALLERGY?

*Exactly what constitutes an allergy is fraught with controversy. Health practitioners from different professional backgrounds may mean different things when they use the term.*

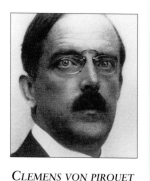

**CLEMENS VON PIRQUET (1874–1924)**
*This Austrian physician coined the term "allergy" in 1906. He used it to describe an abnormal reaction by the body to a normally harmless foreign substance.*

**THE UNLIKELY ENEMY**
*In an allergic reaction normally harmless substances, such as dried cat saliva, can produce damaging immune responses.*

Many people have experienced an allergic reaction—developing a rash after using a new suntan lotion, for instance, or sneezing on entering a damp room. And most hay fever sufferers understand that their symptoms are brought on in the spring or summer by the pollen of certain plants. There are also more subtle kinds of allergic responses, in which symptoms are delayed and seem unrelated to the triggering substance. Some food allergies are examples of such reactions. But why should an apparently harmless substance, like a pollen grain, cause physical problems?

## ALLERGY AND THE IMMUNE SYSTEM

Doctors have learned that in such reactions as hay fever or eczema it is the body's immune system that causes the symptoms. What seems to happen in an allergic reaction is that a substance, like a pollen, that normally would present no threat to the body is seen as hostile by the immune system. The "invader" is expelled by sneezing, coughing, a runny nose, or a weeping rash.

To properly understand what an allergy is, a basic understanding of the immune system—its components and how they work together—is essential. The role of the immune system is to protect us from potentially harmful substances and organisms that could cause disease or infection. It is composed of several different types of cells present in blood and tissues, especially in parts of the body that are exposed to the external environment—the eyes and nose, for example. These cells are able to recognize hostile organisms or foreign material and retaliate by producing defensive weapons directed specifically at the invaders.

### Antibodies and immune cells

Antibodies are the "foot-soldiers" of the immune system. Their job is to recognize and identify foreign organisms and substances, attack them directly, and interact with other cells in the immune system to destroy invaders. A newborn baby is equipped with some antibodies from its mother, but most are produced after birth.

Antibodies, found in the blood and other body fluids, are proteins whose structure is precisely engineered to fit the surface components of germs, like a key fits into a lock. Antibodies are more precisely termed immunoglobulins (abbreviated Ig) and are divided into subclasses that are identified as IgA, IgD, IgE, IgG, and IgM.

Each class of antibody works in a somewhat different way and has a different job to do. Some cause the release of large numbers of chemical messengers; others bind to the target germs and cause them to clump together. The larger clumps then attract white blood cells, such as phagocytes, that engulf and digest them.

IgE antibodies are especially important in allergic reactions. They coat mast cells and basophils (types of immune cells), acting as receptors—molecules on the surface of a cell that recognize and bind to passing molecules and trigger changes inside the cell.

When an invading allergen (any substance, particle, or organism that provokes an allergic response) binds to IgE receptors, the mast cells or basophils release their cargo of inflammatory messenger chemicals, such as histamine, thus triggering

## ELEMENTS OF THE IMMUNE SYSTEM

The immune system is composed of cells whose function is to identify, attack, and destroy invaders. However, each of these soldier elements can be triggered by harmless substances as well as germs. When this happens, and allergic symptoms result, the reaction is called allergy, as opposed to immunity.

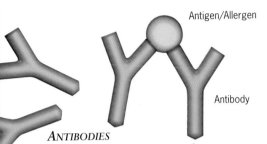

Antigen/Allergen

Antibody

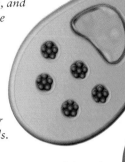

### ANTIBODIES
*These complex proteins are the main-stay of the immune system. Each antibody is specific for a particular target substance, called an antigen, or allergen.*

### LYMPHOCYTES
*There are several varieties of lymphocytes, including B- and T-cells. They are important in initiating immune responses, and have many other functions as well. For instance, T-cells have the ability to destroy foreign cells.*

### MAST CELLS AND BASOPHILS
*These are found in the skin, mucous membranes, and blood. Mast cells are fixed in position, while basophils circulate freely in the blood. Both types contain granules of histamine and other messenger chemicals.*

T-cell

B-cell

Mast cell

Basophil

Polymorph

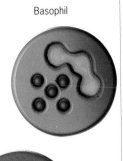

### PHAGOCYTES
*Polymorphs and macrophages—collectively called phagocytes—are cells that crawl around the body like amoebas, engulfing and digesting such microscopic particles as germs, thus removing them and preventing them from doing harm.*

---

inflammation. The inflammation brings immune cells into the area, provides the optimal temperature for their activity, and flushes the affected tissue with fluid to help wash away germs or allergens and the debris of cell damage.

Besides the phagocytes, which overwhelm smaller allergens and germs, other significant cells in the immune system are the lymphocytes. These are the heavy artillery, which may be called upon to help fight particularly resistant infections. They can initiate immune responses and attack foreign cells directly. One type of lymphocyte, known as B-cells, can turn into antibody factories, secreting various types of immunoglobulin into the blood.

Complement is the name given to another group of proteins in normal blood that can be activated during an immune reaction to combine with antibodies and help kill bacteria and other invading cells. Once activated, they also serve to induce inflammation.

Although the list above is by no means a complete accounting of the immune system, it covers the elements essential to the production of an allergic reaction.

### THE PHYSIOLOGY OF AN ALLERGY
The different forces of the immune system outlined above are marshaled into several lines of defense. Where tissues are in direct contact with the outside world—the skin,

## THE LYMPHATIC SYSTEM

The lymphatic system is an important part of the body's immune system. It consists of a set of vessels that collect lymph fluid from the tissues of the body and drain it back into the blood. Lymph nodes, situated throughout the lymphatic system, act as a barrier to the spread of infection by destroying or filtering out bacteria and other harmful agents.

### LYMPH FLUID
*Lymph is a clear fluid composed of water, protein, and sundry other substances. It carries white blood cells, which help fight infections.*

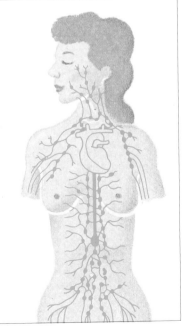

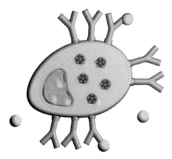

**Step 1** IgE antibodies adhere to receptors on the membrane of a mast cell, each of which is specific to one allergen.

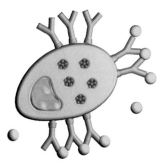

**Step 2** The antibodies react with the allergens, activating the mast cell.

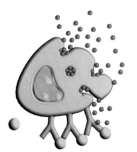

**Step 3** The mast cell degranulates, releasing its cargo of inflammatory chemicals.

and the respiratory and intestinal tracts—various elements of the immune system are concentrated. For instance, mast cells and basophils are anchored in the connective tissues of the skin and the lining of the lungs; phagocytes patrol in the blood, the mucus of the sinuses, and tear ducts of the eyes; and antibodies can be found almost everywhere in the body.

If an allergen is seen as a risk by the immune system—for example when a bee injects venom into the skin or pollen gets into the mucus of the lungs—one or more elements of the immune system recognizes the invading substance or some part of it as a hostile entity. This sets in motion a train of events that may include the release of chemical messengers, such as histamine or heparin, the activation of the complement, or the attack of killer T-cells. This will not happen on the first encounter with an allergen because the immune system needs at least one exposure to become sensitized to a specific allergen.

Immunologists recognize four types of immune response to allergens. Each is defined in terms of the mechanism involved, rather than the symptoms produced.

## Type I allergy

A Type I allergy is caused mostly by antibodies of the IgE class, which are found on the surfaces of basophils and mast cells. When these antibodies recognize the precise antigen they were made for and bind to it, histamine and other inflammatory substances are released from the cells. The result is an inflammation in which reddening and itchiness are the major features.

IgE antibodies appear to have few beneficial effects, except perhaps for helping to rid the body of worms and other parasites, which are not a major problem in the developed world. When Type I allergy affects the moist membranes of the eyes, nose, lungs, or intestines, it produces mucus (runny nose, phlegm) and involuntary expulsive efforts (sneezing, coughing, vomiting, or scratching, depending on which organ is affected). This type of reaction matches most closely with what environmental allergists, or clinical ecologists, term Type A allergy (see page 20).

Type I allergy is also known as atopy. An individual is said to be atopic when he or she overproduces IgE. This means that IgE is at a raised level in the blood and on mast

## INFLAMMATION

Inflammation is the body's natural response to invaders or foreign substances that have not been fully dealt with by the immune system and have started to cause damage. Inflammation is recognizable by its five cardinal signs: swelling of the area, redness, heat, pain, and impaired function. Histamine and other chemical messengers cause the capillaries—tiny blood vessels in the skin—to dilate, stretching their walls so that fluid and immune cells leak into the surrounding tissues and deal with the invaders.

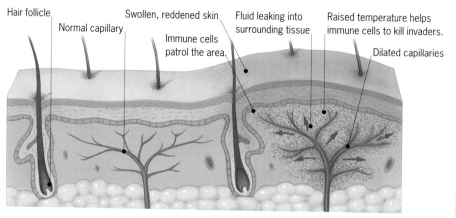

**Skin without inflammation** exhibits normal color and temperature. There are no unusual raised areas, swelling, or unusual immune activity.

**Inflamed skin** is reddened and the surface is warm. Leaky capillaries cause swelling as fluid builds up. Immune cells patrol the area.

cells, so that the sufferer is always reactive to even low levels of whatever allergen stimulated the antibody production in the first place—for instance mold spores, chemicals, pollen, or house dust, which are constantly present in the atmosphere.

As a result, sufferers have an allergic reaction, such as asthma, eczema, urticaria (itching), or rhinitis, whenever they are exposed to the allergen, which may be a seasonal occurrence or may happen constantly. A classic example would be hay fever, in which allergy to airborne pollen grains causes the eyes and nose to become inflamed (conjunctivitis and rhinitis).

## Type II allergy

Type II allergy is caused by antibodies of the IgG or IgM class when they combine with complement to kill antigenic cells (cells that the immune system sees as invaders). One example is drug-induced anemia, which occurs when a particular drug binds to the surface of the patient's red blood cells and causes them to become antigenic, so that the immune system regards them as foreign. This event leads to the production of antibodies, which are called autoantibodies because they are directed against the body's own cells rather than foreign cells. These antibodies are actually directed against the drug molecules stuck to the cells' surfaces, but the effect nonetheless is to activate complement, which causes the red blood cells to break up and results in anemia. A Type II allergy is rare.

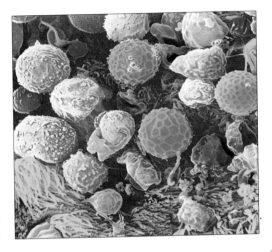

*RESPIRATORY INVADERS*
*Minute particles, like the pollen, dust, and mold spores shown here, can build up in the lungs of people whose jobs expose them to such substances as damp, moldy hay or flour. After prolonged exposure, a Type III allergic reaction can cause a condition like farmer's lung.*

## Type III allergy

Type III allergy is also caused by IgG or IgM antibodies and complement, but the damage is caused by the inflammatory action of complement. The inflammation develops more slowly than in Type I inflammation and lasts longer. The affected area does not itch much but is very tender. The classic example of a Type III reaction would be farmer's lung, caused by the inhalation of fungal spores during the handling of damp hay, which causes inflammation of the lungs. Occupational exposure to mold spores also causes cheese washer's disease, furrier's lung, and maple bark stripper's lung.

## Type IV allergy

Type IV allergy is caused not by antibodies but by lymphocytes of the kind known as killer cells. These cells can kill any invading microorganisms externally, without having

## CYTOTOXIC T-CELL ATTACK

A type of lymphocyte called cytotoxic T-cell, or killer T-cell, can destroy invaders too large to be ingested by phagocytes. Cytotoxic T-cells are able to recognize and lock on to invading cells, releasing potent enzymes into the fluid surrounding the target, or injecting them directly into it. Killer T-cells are especially important in dealing with Type IV reactions.

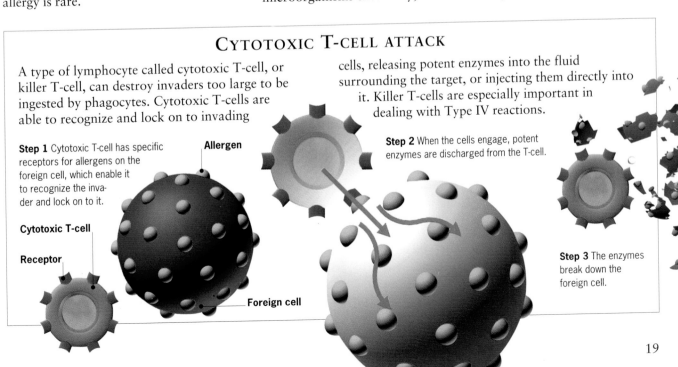

**Step 1** Cytotoxic T-cell has specific receptors for allergens on the foreign cell, which enable it to recognize the invader and lock on to it.

**Allergen**

**Cytotoxic T-cell**

**Receptor**

**Foreign cell**

**Step 2** When the cells engage, potent enzymes are discharged from the T-cell.

**Step 3** The enzymes break down the foreign cell.

## A DIFFERENCE OF APPROACH

Allergists look at whether a patient has IgE antibodies to certain allergens, advise avoidance of triggers, and use medications to control symptoms.

Environmental doctors use many of the same approaches as allergists but consider a wider range of symptoms as indicative of allergies.

**CONVENTIONAL**
*The history of a patient's symptoms plus blood and skin prick tests are used to confirm an allergy, but usually only Type I, involving IgE. Avoidance, immunotherapy, and drugs will be prescribed according to findings.*

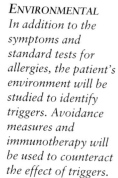

**ENVIRONMENTAL**
*In addition to the symptoms and standard tests for allergies, the patient's environment will be studied to identify triggers. Avoidance measures and immunotherapy will be used to counteract the effect of triggers.*

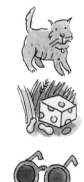

to ingest them first. A Type IV reaction can result in scarring, if severe enough. A classic example of a mild Type IV allergy is contact allergy to the nickel in some jewelery. Type IV responses can also cause other types of hypersensitive reactions, involving diseases like tuberculosis and leprosy.

### DIFFERENT SCHOOLS OF THOUGHT

Allergists fall generally into one of two schools: conventional and environmental, also known as clinical ecologists. They differ primarily over the issue of what constitutes an allergic reaction and what does not. But this dispute also leads to disagreements on questions such as which substances can act as allergens and which health conditions are the result of allergies.

### The conventional approach

Conventional allergists and clinical ecologists both agree that reactions that do not have an immunological mechanism are not allergies. But conventional allergists go further. They hold that any condition that has not been clearly shown to conform to one of the four types of mechanism is not an allergy. It is not unusual for patients who are found to be negative for Type I allergy to be told that their problems are not due to allergic reactions. Even in the strictest scientific terms this may not be true because a lot of work is still needed to establish—or rule out—the involvement of the Types II, III,

and IV mechanisms, and most of the tests that conventional allergists consider reliable enough to use apply only to Type I allergies.

### The environmental approach

Practitioners of environmental medicine and clinical ecologists (see pages 46—47) start by establishing that environmental influences make the patient ill and that avoiding exposure can make a substantial difference to their well-being. This occurs in two patterns that they refer to as Type A and intolerance. However, because many cases referred to as intolerance have features that are suggestive of immunological mechanisms, clinical ecologists may call them Type B allergies.

### TYPE A AND TYPE B ALLERGIES

Generally speaking, Type A allergies include most of the forms recognized by immunologists, for instance, hay fever. Type B allergies show some characteristics of immune reactions, for instance they are specific to particular allergens and they may eventually be shown to result from Type III or IV mechanisms. But unlike Type A symptoms, they often have delayed effects or they affect other parts of the body. For example, inhaling pollen could lead to gut pains, aching joints, or eczema, none of which are symptoms typically associated with a pollen allergy. Or an allergy to a food might cause symptoms in a part of the body not associated with the mouth or gut—nasal symptoms, like rhinitis, for instance. The symptoms might take several hours to develop, and if the food is eaten often it will never be clear that there is a link between eating the food and the onset of nasal symptoms. Both of these examples would be considered Type B reactions.

## Intolerance

Other types of reaction are intolerances due to a shortage of enzymes or to chronic toxicity. These are not allergies. Since it is not always easy to differentiate between allergy and intolerance, however, some people refer to Type B reactions as intolerances. Conventional allergists argue that intolerance and other nonallergic mechanisms underlie most Type B reactions. Clinical ecologists disagree, and this is the source of some of the most bitter controversy in the field.

## Other types of reactions

Symptoms that closely resemble those of Type A or Type B can also be produced by other nonallergic reactions, such as chronic toxicity or pseudoallergy. Alternative practitioners sometimes use the term "allergy" more loosely to include such reactions. In fact, conditions in real life may not be clear cut, often containing elements of several different phenomena.

## Strengths and weaknesses

The differences between conventional allergists and clinical ecologists arise, in part, because the former base their classification mainly on underlying mechanisms rather than symptoms, while the latter use symptoms and their response to treatment, more often than mechanisms, as a guide. Also, conventional allergists rely on laboratory findings for diagnosis, while there are no simple laboratory tests for a Type B allergy. The ranges of the symptoms differ too.

Both systems of classification have their strengths and weaknesses. Unfortunately, environmental approaches have few double-blind tests to back them up; they are based largely on anecdotal evidence and some of their practitioners have "discovered" allergies in up to 90 percent of their patients.

While conventional allergists have more science on their side, they tend not to heed sensitivities that do not involve the immune system and may dismiss very real illnesses. Doctors of the clinical ecology school are less concerned with the biological mechanisms involved and more interested in what happens to patients when suspect items are eliminated and then reintroduced, or the environment is altered in the home or workplace.

## Masked allergy

In particular, the environmental medicine approach recognizes a condition called masked allergy, which conventional allergists do not acknowledge. Some practitioners argue that certain forms of masked allergy are actually a type of food addiction. (See Chapter 4 for more details.)

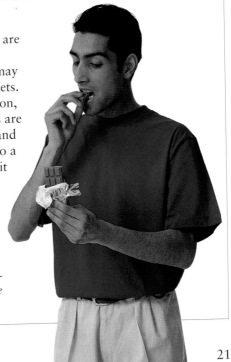

## FOOD ADDICTION

Addictions to certain foods are quite common and are not restricted, as some people may believe, to caffeine and sweets. Any food can cause addiction, but the commonest culprits are milk, wheat, cheese, nuts, and chocolate. Being addicted to a food means that removing it from the diet can provoke withdrawal symptoms.

*PRIME SUSPECTS*
*Foods that elicit strong feelings—and these include both cravings and aversions—should be considered as prime suspects in food allergy.*

# CONTROVERSY IN THE WORLD OF ALLERGIES

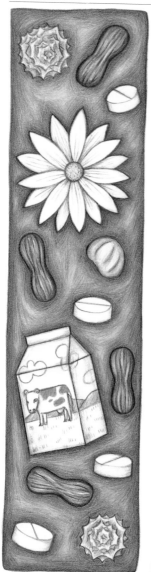

Allergist/immunologists and clinical ecologists disagree over several issues and use the term "allergy" differently. Immunologists use allergy to mean an immune-mediated reaction, while clinical ecologists use it to mean the harmful effect of an environmental or dietary substance, which has features indicating that it may be caused by an immunological reaction. The latter group classifies allergies on the basis of clinical pattern, while the former uses the four types of immunological reaction. Allergists restrict the list of conditions that they consider allergies to such reactions as hay fever, asthma, and eczema, whereas clinical ecologists include all of these, as well as arthritis, migraine, weight fluctuation, hyperactivity, irritable bowel syndrome, and other conditions. Immunologists look for allergies using defined tests, but clinical ecologists have no reliable laboratory diagnostic methods. Both groups advocate the avoidance of allergens. Immunologists also use drug treatment to prevent and/or alleviate symptoms, while environmental allergists avoid drugs whenever possible.

| CONTROVERSIAL AREA | ALLERGIST/IMMUNOLOGISTS | CLINICAL ECOLOGISTS |
| --- | --- | --- |
| Meaning of "allergy" | Immune-mediated reaction (i.e. caused by the action of the immune system) | Sensitivity to an environmental or dietary substance with features that suggest allergy |
| Classification of allergies | Types I–IV immunology | Types A and B, based on the pattern of symptoms and response to avoidance |
| What conditions might be considered allergic | Hay fever, asthma, eczema, urticaria, anaphylaxis | All standard allergies plus others, including mood disorders and hidden food allergies |
| Methods of diagnosis | Scratch or skin-prick test, RAST, challenge test | Cytotoxic test, kinesiology, IgG ELISA test, pulse rate changes. Diagnosis is sometimes based only on a patient's history. |
| Methods of treatment | Avoidance of allergen, drug treatments, immunotherapy for pollen, dust mites, and venom allergies | Avoidance of allergen or desensitization to a wider range of allergens, sublingual immunotherapy |

## ALLERGIC SYMPTOMS

The most familiar allergic symptoms are those that environmental allergists would classify as Type A; they tend to be short, intense, and discrete in onset and effect. Type B symptoms are more likely to be chronic and vague, and they often appear to be unconnected with the trigger or triggers.

## Type A symptoms

Most people are familiar with the classic symptoms of well-known conditions, such as hay fever or peanut allergy. The systems affected by these are the body's most vulnerable—the skin and the respiratory and gastrointestinal systems.

Sneezing, coughing, and excessive production of mucus causing a runny nose and phlegm are obvious characteristics of Type A allergies. A more severe problem is asthma, in which the airways constrict and become filled with mucus, making breathing difficult (see page 72). Asthma ranges in severity and is sometimes fatal. It is becoming more common, particularly among children and young adults. Some children grow out of it. Eye problems—allergic conjunctivitis—including itching, swelling, and watering, are common Type A symptoms, especially with an allergy to animals.

Foods and antibiotics often cause gastrointestinal problems, such as vomiting, diarrhea, or abdominal pain. In Type A conditions these symptoms come on almost immediately. They may also be accompanied by skin problems, like eczema or hives. The immediacy of effect makes it relatively easy to identify the trigger.

Eczema, or dermatitis, may be a Type A reaction. Initially there is an increased blood flow to the affected area, causing redness. This is followed by itchiness and the formation of blisters, which may rupture and weep. The skin becomes thickened and flaky, and the condition may become chronic.

Urticaria, also called nettle rash or hives, involves swelling and discoloration of the skin. The swelling can be either deep-seated or superficial. The latter is common in Type A allergies, and although usually acute and short-lived, it can be very irritating. Deeper swelling, known as angioedema, is often associated with allergenic foods and is mostly restricted to the face, lips, tongue, and throat. Angioedema comes on very quickly, sometimes immediately.

## Anaphylaxis

Anaphylaxis is a rare but potentially life-threatening condition that results from extreme sensitivity to an allergen. In a strictly clinical sense, anaphylaxis refers to any sort of hypersensitive reaction and can be local and relatively mild. However, the term usually is used to mean anaphylactic shock, which is a system-wide reaction.

The most common causes of anaphylaxis are peanuts, tree nuts, seafood, wasp and bee venom, and antibiotics like penicillin. The effects are rapid, with itching and all-over swelling, wheezing, a dangerous drop in blood pressure, and possibly heart failure. A few cases every year are fatal, but normally anaphylactic shock is not this severe and responds well to prompt treatment.

Anaphylaxis usually involves IgE antibodies in a Type I reaction, but there are alternative routes, such as the activation of complement or nonimmune pathways that mimic anaphylaxis. These are called anaphylactoid reactions and respond to the same sort of treatment (see Chapter 7).

## Chronic symptoms

Many immunologists and other conventional doctors dismiss the claims that Type B allergies can cause a wide range of chronic disorders and symptoms. This dismissal is easier to understand when the number of symptoms and the disorders with which they be associated is considered. Many of the symptoms, such as sleeplessness or excessive sweating, are vague and hard to pin down. Nonetheless, they pose a real problem for sufferers, who may be misdiagnosed or dismissed as hypochondriac.

Doctors even have a name for what they see as a basically psychological condition—somatization disorder. Fortunately these symptoms sometimes respond well to an environmental treatment—namely, avoidance of the trigger—and the exact cause, or allergen, may not have to be identified for treatment to be effective.

### Symptoms of Type B conditions

Type B conditions can involve a wide range of disorders that affect almost every system in the body. These include fatigue and lethargy; heartburn; sleeplessness; catarrh and sinus problems; cold hands and feet; constant runny nose; diarrhea or constipation (or both); sore lips, gums, eyes, and tongue; weight fluctuation, bloating, or obesity; chronic gas or indigestion; skin and hair problems; migraine and other headaches; muscle, joint, and bone aches; arthritis; excessive sweating; hyperactivity; cystitis; depression and irritability; stress incontinence; asthma; and menstrual problems.

## SYMPTOMS OF TYPES A AND B REACTIONS

There are key differences between the symptoms of Type A and Type B allergic reactions. While most Type A symptoms occur immediately and are localized,

Type B reactions may be delayed, and they often occur elsewhere in the body, leading to problems that are much harder to diagnose.

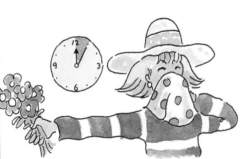

**IMMEDIATE**
*Type A symptoms tend to appear at or near the point of contact with an allergen—for example, swollen eyes or sneezing.*

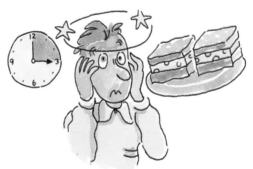

**DELAYED**
*Type B symptoms, such as migraine, may appear soon after contact with an allergen, but often take hours or days to develop.*

# COMMON ALLERGENS

*Any substance that causes an allergic reaction is termed an "allergen." There are thousands of known allergens, of which a few dozen are particularly notorious troublemakers.*

Virtually any substance can cause an allergy. However, all allergens can be put on a scale that ranges from very common to quite rare.

### WHAT MAKES A SUBSTANCE ALLERGENIC?

To a large extent the frequency with which a substance causes an allergy depends on how much of it there is in our lives. Cow's milk heads the list of foods causing Type B allergies, probably because it is encountered so early in life, and in the Western world it is widely consumed by adults, almost every day. But milk allergy is extremely rare in China, where very few adults consume it because of their genetic inability to digest lactose, the sugar found in milk.

### The people factor

The way in which allergies have emerged as a problem over the past 200 years suggests that another factor—something in the modern environment—is important in determining how individuals respond to allergens. Since the Industrial Revolution there has

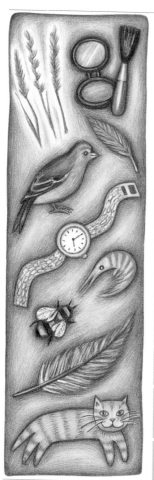

## COMMON ALLERGENS

Allergens can be categorized by their route of contact and by their biological or chemical nature. In the table below the most common allergens are divided into the most useful groupings frequently used in diagnosis and treatment. As the table shows, some allergens that cause Type A reactions can also cause Type B.

| NATURE OF ALLERGEN | ROUTE OF CONTACT | ALLERGENS CAUSING TYPES A AND B REACTIONS | ALLERGENS CAUSING TYPE B REACTIONS |
|---|---|---|---|
| Aeroallergens | Inhaled | Grass pollens, tree and plant pollens, dust mites, mold spores, wool fibers, feathers, some chemicals | Inhaled chemical pollutants and volatile organic chemicals (VOCs) |
| Food | Ingested or on contact | Mainly milk, shellfish, fish, wheat, soy, eggs, peanuts, tree nuts | All foods, especially those eaten frequently, such as milk products and wheat food additives such as colorings, flavorings, and preservatives; food contaminants |
| Animal | Inhaled or on contact | Dogs, cats, horses, rabbits, guinea pigs, birds | |
| Biting/ stinging insects | Bites or stings | Wasps, bees, mosquitoes, hornets, horseflies | |
| Drugs | Ingested, injected, or applied | Various, antibiotics in particular | Many drugs and their fillers; colorings and preservatives |
| Other | On contact | Latex, nickel and other metals, semen, makeup | |

been a vast increase in the levels of synthesized and polluting chemicals that we breathe, eat, and drink. In industrial countries there has been a marked increase in both Type A and Type B allergy symptoms over the past 50 years, and levels are rising in less developed countries as they become industrialized. It certainly seems as if there could be a a link between environmental change and allergies in general (see Chapter 3 for more details). However, such a link does not explain which substances cause problems and why.

## The raw and the cooked
Several factors determine whether a food will cause problems. In particular, certain foods change their allergenic properties, depending on how they are prepared.

Cooking can change the reactive properties of some foods for the better. For example, soaking and cooking beans destroys toxins in them that can cause digestive problems, and some allergens in milk are broken down when heated. Milk is also altered during the process of making cheese, yogurt, or butter, and some people who cannot drink milk can tolerate these foods. On the other hand, processed and manufactured foods nearly always contain a host of colorings, flavorings, and preservatives that can trigger allergic reactions in many people.

## Allergens as toxins
Sometimes an allergen has toxic effects as well as ones that are antigenic (causing an immune reaction). Even pollen grains and dust mites, the classic "harmless" allergens, are capable of bursting open and killing red blood cells if placed close to them, and the toxins responsible are inflammatory to human skin. Clearly toxicology is important as well as immunology, but this is a controversial area about which little is known.

## Understanding allergic symptoms
How can we start to make sense of the apparently senseless inflammation, the "immunity gone wrong," that constitutes Type I allergy? Sneezing, coughing, vomiting, and diarrhea are all obvious excretion mechanisms, as is the outpouring of mucus that accompanies them. Eczema and urticaria, the itchy components, may also enhance excretion from the skin because the scratching that ensues encourages lymph

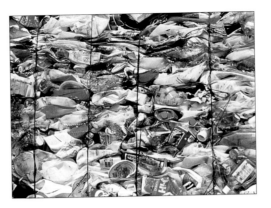

flow and perhaps excretion of trigger substances through the skin itself in the weeping fluid of eczema. Asthma, which restricts air intake into the lungs, will prevent entry of allergenic particles and germs and encourage turbulent air flow in breathing out, which in turn increases the passage of mucus out of the lungs.

In this view, Type A allergic symptoms represent the body's attempts (usually successful) to expel potentially harmful gases and particles from the body. Type B symptoms could be taken as a sign that these attempts have been ineffective, that the body's defense systems have been overwhelmed or were not strong enough in the first place. Why does this happen and what can be done about it? The answers are urgently needed because the incidence of Type B allergic conditions is growing fast. These questions cannot be answered fully at present, but improved nutrition and lessened exposure to chemicals might help to slow this rise, particularly in the very young.

None of this means that doctors should not try to treat and alleviate allergic symptoms. But it should dictate a note of caution in therapy. Itching and wheezing may be doing a useful job, so rather than exert efforts to suppress symptoms, it may be better to seek the underlying causes of their provocation.

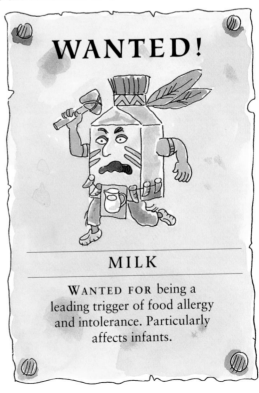

**WANTED!**

MILK

WANTED FOR being a leading trigger of food allergy and intolerance. Particularly affects infants.

# WHO GETS ALLERGIES AND WHY?

*Although genetics play a part in susceptibility to allergies, they can be hard to separate from the role played by environmental factors, particularly around the time of birth.*

*ARE ALLERGIES HEREDITARY?*
*Type I allergies—the most well understood ones—tend to run in families, though the genetics are complex and have not yet been fully worked out.*

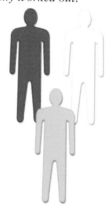

**A person with one atopic parent** (see Glossary) has about a 35 percent chance of developing Type I allergies.

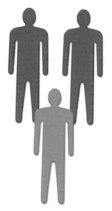

**If both parents are atopic,** the probability of developing such allergies is about 70 percent.

Biological characteristics are determined by a combination of genetic and environmental factors, and allergies are no exception. While scientists have investigated how allergies develop, much on this subject remains obscure. It is definitely known that having an immune system sensitive to normally harmless substances is partly a matter of heredity, particularly with Type I allergy, or atopy. But many studies have also shown that there is a "window of vulnerability" during the months just before and after birth, when a susceptible individual can become sensitized to allergens. Sensitization can happen throughout life, but it becomes less likely with advancing age. Environmental factors interact with a genetic predisposition to determine the final extent and severity of an individual's allergies.

### HOW COMMON ARE ALLERGIES?

Estimates vary about the incidence of allergies, depending on which conditions are considered to be allergic, but the most conservative estimate is that asthma, eczema, and hay fever affect 10 to 20 percent of the population. If the conditions classified as Type B were to be included, this estimate would more than double.

American allergist William Rea suggests that allergy patients who go to see doctors represent the tip of a very large iceberg, and that mild degrees of allergic illness are so common that only very few people are completely well and functioning at full potential. Certainly, experienced allergists see mild cases all around them among family and friends. As the famous English physician Richard Asher put it, "Allergists see the world through allergy-colored spectacles."

It seems probable that the health of many people could be improved by careful attention to diet and environment.

### Twins

In pairs of identical twins, one may have a severe Type I allergic illness and the other may not, even though the unaffected twin has positive IgE and skin tests. This indicates that factors other than heredity are at work. Once an individual has the genetic potential to become allergic, one or more environmental factors may be needed to trigger the development of an allergy.

### Infant exposure

The first few weeks of life are crucial. If babies are kept away from dust, furry animals, and common allergenic foods during this time, they are less likely to develop Type I allergies in later years. The mother should avoid eating the same things over

### NATURE OR NURTURE?

Children inherit far more than genes from their parents; they also inherit dietary and lifestyle habits. This fact makes it hard for scientists studying the genetics of allergy to figure out the extent to which susceptibility to allergies is determined by genes and the extent to which it depends on a person's environment, particularly their early environment. For instance, conditions in the womb are vital in determining allergies, but these conditions depend to some degree on the mother's genes.

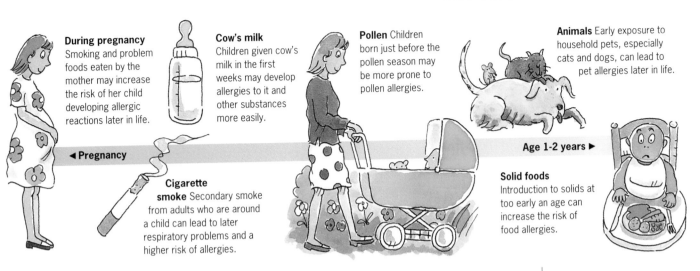

**During pregnancy** Smoking and problem foods eaten by the mother may increase the risk of her child developing allergic reactions later in life.

**Cow's milk** Children given cow's milk in the first weeks may develop allergies to it and other substances more easily.

**Pollen** Children born just before the pollen season may be more prone to pollen allergies.

**Animals** Early exposure to household pets, especially cats and dogs, can lead to pet allergies later in life.

◄ **Pregnancy**

**Age 1-2 years ►**

**Cigarette smoke** Secondary smoke from adults who are around a child can lead to later respiratory problems and a higher risk of allergies.

**Solid foods** Introduction to solids at too early an age can increase the risk of food allergies.

and over for the last few months of pregnancy. During the first few months of the baby's life, the child should be fed nothing other than mother's milk. Breast-fed infants fed solid foods as well develop as many allergies as bottle-fed babies, if not more.

## Tobacco smoke
This is the number one allergy trigger, especially during infancy. Tobacco smoke tends to divert the immune system into IgE production, so dusts, pollens, and foods that the baby encounters during the first months are more likely to cause trouble later if he or she is exposed to smoke at the same time.

## Cow's milk
There is some evidence that cow's milk can make a child more likely to react to other allergens. Allergists tend to be suspicious of milk, in spite of its nutritional value, because it so often acts as an allergen itself, causing numerous childhood health problems. However milk and milk products are an excellent source of calcium, and children should not be taken off milk unless their nutrition is carefully balanced in other ways.

## Season of birth
Studies show that babies who are born during the spring months at the start of the pollen season are more likely to become allergic to pollens than those born during the winter months. This can probably be attributed to the window of vulnerability during the first few weeks of life.

## Infections and traumas
Symptoms of both Type A and Type B allergies often occur for the first time after a bout of flu or glandular fever. Type B

conditions frequently follow other traumas (physical, chemical, or emotional), especially when these occur closely together.

## Nutrition
Modern fast food of the hamburger and cola variety, although rich in calories and proteins, tends to be poor in important vitamins and trace minerals. Many people do survive this kind of diet without apparent ill effects, but they become more vulnerable to the various triggers listed above, especially if they are genetically predisposed to allergies. There is evidence that patients with allergies are often short of certain nutrients, such as magnesium, but it is unclear whether this is a cause or a result of an allergy.

### HERITABILITY OF INTOLERANCES
Symptoms similar to those of Type B allergy may be caused by intolerances or pseudo-allergies (see page 21). An intolerance—the inability to digest lactose, for instance—can be caused by an enzyme deficiency (see page 78). Such a deficiency could be due in turn to a hereditary genetic factor.

*CHILDHOOD DANGERS*
*Expectant and breast-feeding mothers who have allergies should avoid foods and medications that they themselves are sensitive to. All mothers should be aware of the dangers of introducing babies to potential allergens in the months just before and after birth.*

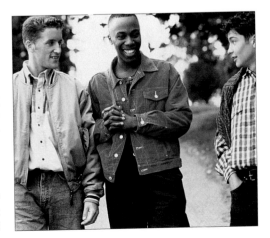

*LACTOSE INTOLERANCE*
*Most people of African and Oriental descent are lactose intolerant as adults (see page 78) because they are genetically programmed to stop producing lactase, the enzyme that breaks down lactose, after infancy.*

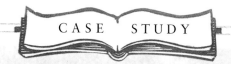

**CASE STUDY**

# A New Allergy Sufferer

*Many allergies develop during early childhood, fade during adolescence and early adulthood, and then reappear in middle or old age. Other allergies simply do not develop until an individual has repeated contact with the allergen. Nickel, for instance, despite being one of the most common causes of contact allergy, may not cause trouble until relatively late in life.*

On her 16th birthday Emily had her ears pierced and was given a pair of gold-colored earrings by a friend at school. Within a few days her ear lobes had become itchy and inflamed. Bathing the wounds in antiseptic at home did not help, so she went to see the family doctor. He diagnosed an infection, told her to stop wearing the earrings, and prescribed a course of antibiotics. However, the drugs did not help much, and the problem with her ears did not clear up. Over the next few weeks she developed patches of itchy, dry skin, similar to those on her ear lobes, elsewhere on her body—the insides of her elbows and knees, for example, and particularly on her wrists and in the middle of her back.

## WHAT SHOULD EMILY DO?

When Emily visited her doctor again he realized that his first diagnosis had probably been wrong and decided to refer her to an allergy specialist (see page 34). The specialist did a skin test to confirm his suspicions that Emily was suffering an allergic reaction to nickel, a common component of earrings and piercing needles. He advised Emily to avoid all contact with nickel in order to give her condition a chance to clear up. She should change not only her earrings but also her watch strap, bracelets, and bra clasps, which all contain nickel and have also caused a reaction. Emily must be careful from now on when handling change and choosing jewelery and clothing.

### HEALTH
*Allergic reactions to contact with an allergen can cause eczema, in which the skin is flaky and itchy and develops a rash.*

### CLOTHING
*Metal costume jewelery frequently contains nickel, and it is sometimes an element in silver, gold (both yellow and white), and platinum. It is also found in metal fittings like buttons and clasps.*

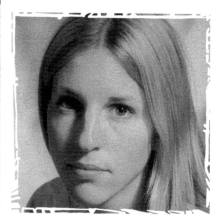

### LIFESTYLE
*Nickel is a very common cause of contact allergy for women, mainly as a result of ear piercing.*

---

## Action Plan

### HEALTH
*Avoid contact with anything that contains nickel to help clear up the allergic reaction. (Emily might have avoided becoming sensitized to nickel if she had realized that piercing can be done with nickel-free steel needles and had not worn earrings containing nickel.)*

### POSSESSIONS
*Become more conscious about the content of buttons and other fasteners on clothing and her way of handling anything metallic, such as touching change with sweaty hands. Wear only sterling silver or 18-carat gold jewelery.*

---

## HOW THINGS TURNED OUT FOR EMILY

The allergist told her that she had allergic contact eczema, rather than an infection, and advised her on how to avoid nickel completely, for instance, by wearing sterling silver, 18-carat gold, or nickel-free steel earrings. She bought a leather watch strap and bras with plastic fastenings and got rid of some costume jewelery she had bought as a child. Within a few weeks, Emily's eczema had cleared up and her skin had returned to normal.

# ALLERGY AND OTHER ILLNESSES

*Allergic reactions have complicated short- and long-term effects on many systems of the body. Naturally, such effects interact with and are affected by other diseases and disorders.*

Conventional medicine maintains what many allergy specialists consider to be an artificial divide between allergies and illnesses. The list of Type B symptoms includes a range of disorders normally considered to be nonallergic, but these disorders respond to conventional treatment for allergies and seem to be similar to allergies in other significant ways. To confuse matters further, there can be a great deal of cause and effect between allergic and nonallergic conditions. Allergy symptoms can be exacerbated, or even provoked, by illnesses and as vice versa. This synergy can make it hard to determine what is causing the particular problem.

## Type A illnesses

Type A reactions may be caused exclusively by a Type A allergy, but sometimes a Type B allergy and other factors play a part. In some cases of eczema, for example, the underlying problem is an allergy to dust mites, which causes an itch. But the rash may not appear until the patient scratches. Once the skin has been abraded by scratching, bacteria can easily set up an infection. There can also be an indirect influence on an allergic disorder. For instance, stress can aggravate eczema, in part because under stress an itch becomes more irritating and causes the patient to scratch more, and partly because stress changes the immune sys-

tem's reaction to allergic triggers (see page 41). Also, deficiencies of some nutrients affect most allergies, particularly eczema.

## Food allergies and intolerances

Apart from eating certain foods frequently, the factors that contribute to the development of Type B food allergy are not well understood. The role of gut flora (bacteria and single-celled organisms that live inside our intestines) in food allergy and intolerance has received a lot of attention recently. There is evidence that levels of yeast, such as Candida, and other organisms, such as Giardia, are important in irritable bowel syndrome and other disorders, and that severe digestive upsets—diarrhea, for instance—can somehow weaken the gut and make it too sensitive (see Chapter 4). Antibiotics taken to treat any infection may cause further problems. By killing off normal, healthy gut flora, they can clear the way for overgrowth of damaging organisms and lead to food intolerance.

### ALLERGIES AND HEALTH

Chapter 9 details the enormous variety of conditions that allergies can cause or complicate, ranging from acne to infertility. But leaving the direct effects of allergic reactions

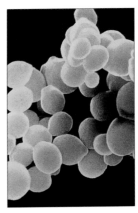

CANDIDA ALBICANS
*Yeast microorganisms like* Candida albicans *are suspected of being involved in a range of Type B conditions, especially gastro-intestinal disorders.*

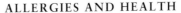

*ITCHY FINGERS*
*Skin allergies often cause itchiness and lead to scratching, which breaks the skin and leaves it vulnerable to infection. To break this chain of events, you can swath the hands of a baby who has eczema in soft mittens.*

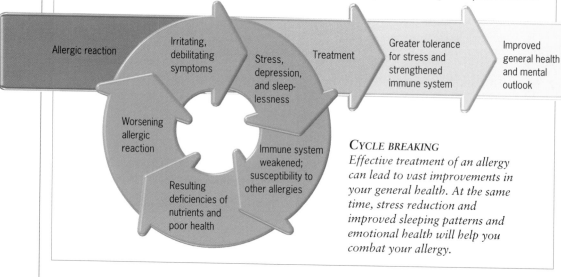

## BREAKING THE CYCLE

An allergic reaction may cause mental and physical stress and set up a worsening cycle of weakened immunity and further allergic reactions. By controlling your symptoms you can break the cycle and improve your health.

Allergic reaction

Irritating, debilitating symptoms

Stress, depression, and sleeplessness

Treatment

Greater tolerance for stress and strengthened immune system

Improved general health and mental outlook

Worsening allergic reaction

Immune system weakened; susceptibility to other allergies

Resulting deficiencies of nutrients and poor health

*CYCLE BREAKING*
*Effective treatment of an allergy can lead to vast improvements in your general health. At the same time, stress reduction and improved sleeping patterns and emotional health will help you combat your allergy.*

aside, what about their indirect effects? It is clear that many allergies can be chronic, or recurrent, in nature, which can have a two-fold effect. First, with the immune system in a constant state of arousal, many of the body's disease-fighting resources will be diverted from more useful pursuits, and at the same time, such essential nutrients as zinc and magnesium will be used up, causing a deficiency. Second, the chronic irritating and debilitating nature of many allergic disorders can eventually take its toll on the psychological health of the individual. Many studies have shown that the mind has a very real and powerful influence on the immune system, and untreated allergies and poor mental health can produce a negative feedback loop.

### Negative feedback
If an allergy sufferer is depressed, stressed, irritable, and losing sleep because of his or her condition, the immune system will suffer accordingly, and the patient's health will get worse. As the body becomes more vulnerable, so it becomes more susceptible to other allergens. Thus a dairy allergy that is left unchecked can lead to the development of sensitivities to other foods. As digestion suffers, so does nutrition, dealing another blow to health. Allergies make general health worse, which in turn worsens the allergies. This is negative feedback.

### Breaking the cycle
Many sufferers of Type B allergies endure constant, grinding misery for years on end, which is why successful treatment can produce such remarkable effects. A careful elimination diet (see Chapters 2 and 4) can break this negative cycle and provide dramatic health gains. The sufferer is relieved from what seemed to be an intractable problem, which doctors either were unable to diagnose or could not treat. Many realize how ill they were only in retrospect.

Recovery from debilitating symptoms starts its own positive feedback loop. Once a person's general health and positive mental outlook are restored, he or she may even be able to start eating some of the foods that used to trigger symptoms.

*FREEDOM FROM ALLERGY MISERY*
*People who have suffered chronic ailments for a long time may discover that a few simple avoidance strategies can transform their lives, enabling them to do things—from walking uphill to sleeping through the night—that were previously beyond them.*

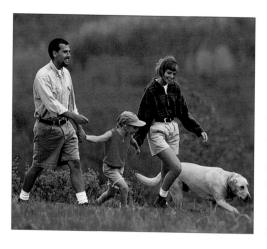

# Nutrient Boosts

*Many nutrients found widely in foods can help protect you against allergies. To function at its best your immune system needs all of these nutrients in the right amounts, and any deficiencies can make you more prone to allergies.*

Given here are some general rules about eating to reduce the risk of allergies, and below are menus that provide an idea of what constitutes a healthful meal plan.

Vary your diet as much as possible and limit the number of times a day you have tea, coffee, and cola or other soft drinks. Drink water more often, preferably bottled or filtered.

Have at least five or six servings a day of fruits and vegetables and vary the types to obtain a wide range of nutrients. Use fresh food as much as possible, to cut down on additives, and choose organic foods when you can, especially if you eat the skins; they are grown without the use of chemical fertilizers and toxic pesticides.

Eat oily fish, such as mackerel, salmon, or sardines, at least once a week and preferably two or three times if possible.

Use a vegetable oil, like safflower, sunflower, or olive, for dressings and cooking and cut down on animal fat.

If you are a vegetarian, make sure you plan your diet to get a sufficient amount of protein.

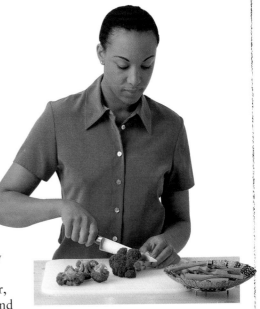

**VEGETABLE NUTRIENT BOOST**
*Eating a selection of fresh vegetables every day supports your immune system.*

## MEAL SUGGESTIONS

### BREAKFAST

► *A bowl of oatmeal and milk or soy milk, topped with banana*

► *Rice cakes topped with a little nut butter and sliced fresh fruit*

### LIGHT MEAL

► *Couscous or rice salad with asparagus, cucumber, and red onion*

► *Turkey or shrimp salad with cucumber, bean sprouts, boiled potatoes, and a selection of greens*

### MAIN MEAL

► *Roast chicken or baked trout with a selection of steamed or roasted vegetables*

► *Baked mackerel with steamed green beans and boiled potatoes*

### DESSERT

► *Sliced fresh fruit, accompanied if you like by soy yogurt*

► *Pancakes made from lentil or millet flour, topped with stewed fruit*

**THE SPICE OF LIFE**
*Fresh ingredients and variety are the keys to a healthy, low-allergen diet.*

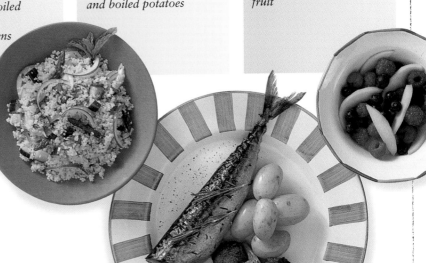

# ALLERGY TESTING

*Pinpointing allergens can be very difficult, and it may be complicated by delayed effects, multiple allergies, and false results. A practitioner's experience is a vital tool in accurate diagnosis.*

Many people do not realize that they are suffering from allergies, especially when foods are involved. Also, the wider implications of allergies and intolerances are still not well understood or accepted by many in the medical profession. This means that if you suspect you have a nonstraightforward allergy, you may have to take the initiative in getting yourself referred and tested. Your doctor may be unaware of the full range of options available, so use this chapter as a very brief guide and research the organizations and services available to you locally.

## PRACTITIONERS
A practitioner's methods of diagnosis and testing will reflect his or her approach to the field as a whole. Immunologists, who restrict their focus to allergy Types I, II, III, and IV, will be interested only in diagnostic methods that test immune response directly, such as measurement of specific antibodies, or in testing for a response that fits the classification, as skin tests do. Environmental allergists also use these methods but look farther afield. They will still want to base their diagnosis on a test that is based on sound scientific principles, such as food challenges or nutritional tests.

Alternative practitioners advocate a range of methods, arguing that as long as a test works and suggests a useful treatment, it does not matter whether its mechanism is understood. This applies to tests like the cytotoxic test (see page 37), Vega (see page 38), or dowsing (see page 36).

## The pros and cons of each approach
The immunological approach has several advantages. Testing is done in controlled situations, so it should be possible to replicate results. Also, because the underlying mechanisms are understood, these tests may provide a better rationale for devising treatment or a better basis for research. The drawbacks of this approach lie in its narrow focus, which really works only for Type I allergies, mostly ignoring Types II, III, and IV, and Type B allergies. Also, even these scientific tests do not give results as reliable as immunologists would like them to.

The tests used by environmental allergists share some of these problems and may also involve a lot of effort. Alternative tests tend not to be supported by rigorous study, and it is hard to verify or assess the claims made for them on strictly scientific grounds.

## Experience counts
Success in testing, in terms of finding the right treatment, depends on the skill and experience of the tester. Alternative tests like dowsing may reflect this, with the dowser's knowledge and experience causing slight movements that lead to diagnosis.

## TESTS
Despite the wide range of tests available, there is only one method that is generally agreed to provide firm diagnostic evidence,

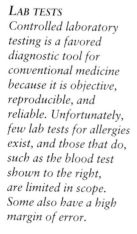

*LAB TESTS*
*Controlled laboratory testing is a favored diagnostic tool for conventional medicine because it is objective, reproducible, and reliable. Unfortunately, few lab tests for allergies exist, and those that do, such as the blood test shown to the right, are limited in scope. Some also have a high margin of error.*

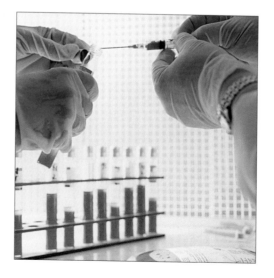

although it is laborious and inconvenient; this is the double-blind challenge. This test can be used for ingestants, as a food challenge, or for inhalants, as a vapor challenge. Skin testing is a sort of contact challenge.

## Challenges

A challenge involves presenting the patient with the suspect allergen to see whether it produces a reaction. If the test is positive several times in a row, the result is unlikely to be a coincidence. Scientists, however, consider that results can be trusted only if the patient does not know which reaction to expect, so that he or she does not imagine or magnify the symptoms.

## Double-blind

The solution is to do the challenges by the "double-blind" method, in which the patient may be presented with either a real test substance or a harmless control, or placebo. Test substances are prepared by a third party so that neither the patient nor the doctor knows which is the real one and can influence the outcome by their various prejudices. If a food is being tested, the challenge might come as a highly flavored stew made with ingredients that are safe for that patient, with the suspect food blended in so that it is undetectable.

The whole process of double-blind testing for allergies is laborious, expensive, and time consuming. A series of appointments must be set up, and some challenges cause symptoms slowly or not at all unless given repeatedly. For pioneer studies on hyperactivity, migraine headaches, and irritable bowel syndrome in the United Kingdom, each challenge had to be administered for two full weeks.

Elaborate double-blind procedures are necessary in rigorous scientific trials, but in practice most environmental allergists find that open food challenges give good enough results to prescribe successful treatments.

## Synergistic factors

A major problem in allergy testing is the role of synergistic factors. These are external factors that can aggravate intolerance—for instance, doing exercise, taking aspirin, drinking alcohol, or being premenstrual. Also, combinations of certain foods can cause reactions, even when each food alone does not. If the relevant synergistic factor is absent, the challenge will be negative even though there is a genuine sensitivity—either an allergy or an intolerance.

This means that although double-blind challenges prove sensitivity when they are positive, they do not disprove it when negative. Sometimes this is not properly understood, and double-blind challenges are interpreted incorrectly to disprove the possibility of sensitivity as a cause of illness.

## Measurement of IgE antibodies (RAST)

Measuring for IgE antibodies in the blood is the standard test for allergies in orthodox medicine. Originally this test was done with

*continued on page 36*

Normally, food elimination diets and subsequent food challenges have to be done over several weeks, leaving plenty of time between each challenge. At special allergy treatment centers careful medical supervision allows patients to go on strict fasts, which clear their systems of allergens. After a fast, patients can then try several food challenges a day, helping to radically speed up identification of trigger foods and substances.

## RAST

RAST (radioallergosorbent test), in which dishes or tubes precoated with specific allergens are used, is widely accepted as the standard laboratory test for Type I allergies. The procedure is easily performed and increasingly reliable. Nonetheless, it is far from perfect and is limited in scope—for instance, it tests only for IgE antibodies, just one of the types involved in allergic reactions.

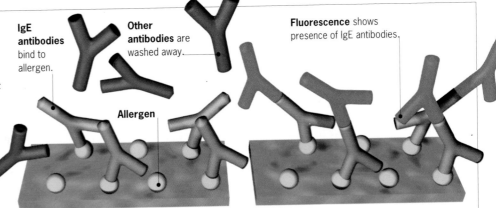

**IgE antibodies** bind to allergen.

**Other antibodies** are washed away.

**Allergen**

**Fluorescence** shows presence of IgE antibodies.

### STEP 1
*Allergens are attached to a dish, and a sample of blood is passed over them then washed off. If IgE antibodies are present, they bind to the allergens.*

### STEP 2
*A special fluorescent antibody is applied, which binds with any bound IgE antibody. Fluorescence shows that the patient has antibodies specific to the test allergen.*

# The Allergist / Immunologist

*Usually the person an allergy sufferer sees after first consulting a primary care physician is a doctor who specializes in allergy and immunology. The allergist uses the basic tools of medicine to identify and help manage allergies.*

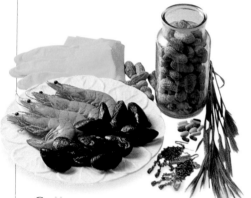

**CLASSICAL ALLERGENS**
*Allergists typically deal with the role of allergens like pollen, nickel, latex, or such common Type A food triggers as milk, eggs, peanuts, tree nuts, and shellfish. These are substances that often provoke Type I allergic reactions.*

Although a primary care physician is trained to recognize when allergy may be a cause of immediate or chronic symptoms, the allergist is the person best equipped to identify what the allergens might be.

**How does the approach of an allergy specialist differ from that of a GP?**
One difference between a general practitioner and an allergist is the amount of time spent on the consultation; few GPs can afford to devote an hour to every new patient, whereas most allergists do just that. Also, an allergist is more aware of the elements in a patient's environment and diet that are likely to trigger allergies, and is better informed in the use of diagnostic methods and treatments for them as well. This specialist has the training and expertise to determine and treat the root causes of an allergic illness, rather than simply suppressing or relieving symptoms.

**What does the training for an allergist/immunologist include?**
An allergist is an M.D.—with a specialty in pediatrics; ear, nose, and throat; or internal medicine—who has an additional two years of postgraduate training in allergy and immunology. In the United States such specialists must pass a certifying examination by the American Board of Allergy and Immunology (ABAI). The Royal College of Physicians and Surgeons is the examining and certification board in Canada.

After becoming certified, an allergist is qualified to diagnose and treat all immune system problems, such as allergies, asthma, immunodeficiency diseases (including AIDS), and autoimmune diseases, like rheumatoid arthritis.

**What can I expect at a consultation?**
All allergy consultations start with a lengthy and detailed history, which can often take an hour or more. The doctor will want to know minute details about the patient's diet, work, and lifestyle, to see if any clues emerge. A patient may have a skin

## Origins

During the 1960s two research teams were seeking the immunoglobin involved in Type I allergic reactions. In 1967 the husband and wife team of Teruko and Kimishige Ishizaka described a new type of immunoglobin—IgE—which they showed was involved in hay fever allergy. Also in 1967 Swedish researchers S. Gunnar O. Johansson and Hans Bennich described the same substance and, in collaboration with another researcher, developed a method for measuring levels of it in blood serum using radioactive particles. This was the radioallergosorbent test, or RAST.

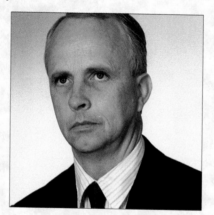

**S. GUNNAR O. JOHANSSON**
*With his partner, Hans Bennich, Johansson identified IgE and developed the RAST.*

rash, for example, that first appeared after using a new dishwashing liquid. Or symptoms may have disappeared during a vacation in the Carribbean, only to reappear on returning home. Once causes are identified, avoidance of them (if possible) is often a matter of common sense. This is why talking is such an essential part of the allergist's procedure, and taking the time to listen to a patient can be excellent therapy in itself.

### What sort of tests will the allergist carry out?

Sometimes the clues are so strong that the specialist stops there and advises a change of diet or lifestyle that may be completely successful. If not, the allergist may do some skin tests or blood tests to obtain more clues. Skin-prick tests usually form the first line of testing, and in many cases RAST (see page 33) may also be used.

The patient may also be asked to keep an accurate diary of everything he or she eats and does, in the hope that unnoticed associations may emerge. If nonallergic conditions could be involved, the specialist will do a physical examination and may also order various tests and X-rays.

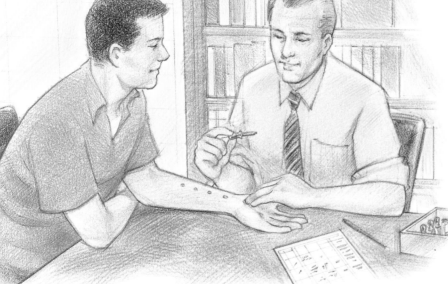

---

## FINDING AN ALLERGIST

In the United States you can contact the American Academy of Allergy, Asthma & Immunology in Milwaukee, Wisconsin. They will send you a list of all the allergists in your area and what their specialties are—for example, animal allergy, pediatric allergy, asthma, rhinitis—as well as their affiliations and certifications. The Asthma and Allergy Foundation of America, headquartered in Washington, D.C., can connect you with other people who are dealing with similar issues and provide information as well.

Most allergists in Canada belong to the Canadian Society of Allergy and Clinical Immunology. To see an allergist you will need a referral from your family doctor, who will send you to one in your area or to the allergy clinic at the nearest hospital.

---

### What treatment might be offered?

Basically the allergist's approach is to devise the best program to help a patient manage allergy, integrating the various forms of conventional treatment available. When it is appropriate, allergists use desensitization because it attacks the root causes of the condition rather than simply suppressing symptoms. This involves periodic injections of increasing amounts of the allergenic extract over a long period, usually one to three years. Some allergists now use one of the newer—and faster—forms of desensitization (see page 48), as evidence for their effectiveness grows, though more studies still need to be conducted.

An allergist also uses medications to relieve symptoms. This is necessary especially when tests fail to pinpoint the allergens, avoidance of them is not possible, or the patient does not have the time or resources to undergo allergy shots.

Hay fever and other pollen allergies are usually treated with drugs that counteract histamines. Most over-the-counter antihistamines cause drowsiness, but prescription drugs are available that are nonsedating. Decongestants may also be given when nasal passages are blocked.

Treatment for asthma includes anti-inflammatory drugs—cromolyn sodium, corticosteroids, or nedocromil—that reduce mucus production and inflammation. (Cromolyn is sometimes advised also as a preventive because it inhibits mast cells from releasing histamine.) Bronchodilators—including beta-agonists and theophylline—are also part of the allergist's arsenal. These are used during an asthma attack to open the airways and make breathing easier. Newer medications, the oral anti-leukotrienes, are also showing promise for treating chronic asthma.

*ALLERGY TESTING*
*An allergist may have a range of allergen samples—for example, pollen extracts—for skin-prick testing. He will select the most likely allergens, based on the pattern and history of a patient's symptoms.*

### Types of skin test

There are three main types of skin test: prick; intracutaneous, or intradermal; and patch. In prick testing, a tiny amount of allergen is introduced into the superficial layer of the skin. For intracutaneous testing, a larger quantity of allergen is injected directly into the dermis. Prick testing is more widely used because it is easier, less expensive and painful, and has less chance of provoking a serious reaction. Intracutaneous tests are slightly more sensitive, and so may be done when a prick test does not give a clear result. Patch tests are used to test reactions to contact with an allergen; they involve attaching some of the test substance to the skin with a plaster to check for a wheal-and-flare response.

radioactive isotopes and was called the radioallergosorbent test, abbreviated to RAST. (Although the radioactive element is no longer used, the name RAST remains.) The advantage of this test is that it gives a precise measurement of specific IgE antibodies in the blood. Its disadvantage is that this reading is only of value with conditions caused by Type I allergy (see page 18). Many doctors have adopted the view that if IgE antibodies are not present, there is no allergy. This view ignores the existence of Type B allergies and allergy Types II through IV.

### Skin tests

For most allergists the first line of physical investigation in addition to RAST is skin-scratch or skin-prick testing, in which tiny volumes of allergen, in liquid form, are introduced into the patient's skin. After 10 minutes or so, if there is specific IgE and the mast cells are sensitive, the skin will blush red, or flare, and produce a raised wheal as a result of the histamine released from the mast cells. This reaction is known as the wheal-and-flare response.

However, the skin mast cells in this particular person may not yield the same reaction as those in the rest of the body. Also, skin tests are not always positive in cases of Type B allergy, although they can detect Type III and Type IV allergies if the skin is observed long enough.

### Basophil and mast cell activation

Simple measurement of blood IgE says nothing about the state of the mast cells and basophils (see page 17), without which IgE cannot do any harm, no matter how much there is. Hence, these tests give a more realistic picture. Basophils are prepared from a blood sample and mixed with the allergen in a test tube. If IgE antibodies are present and if the basophils are susceptible to their effects, the latter undergo various cellular and biochemical changes that can be measured. For instance, when triggered by an allergen, the cell's contents may be released, in a process known as degranulation.

### Dowsing

To conduct this test the practitioner holds a small pendulum over samples of blood or hair from the patient and concentrates on the substance in question. By reading the

> **WARNING**
> *Skin testing is potentially dangerous; occasionally it can cause a severe allergic reaction, such as anaphylactic shock. It should be carried out with due precautions only by an experienced doctor and under close and constant supervision.*

## SKIN-PRICK TEST

Skin testing is one of the key elements in the allergist's diagnostic armoury. The prick test provides a quick, easy, relatively safe method of checking that IgE antibodies are present and reacting with the mast cells in the skin.

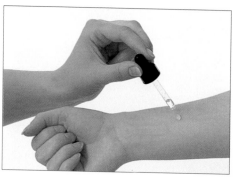

**APPLICATION OF ALLERGEN EXTRACT**
*Usually, a small drop of extract is put on the forearm. Testing sites should be about 2 cm (1 in) apart, in two or three rows.*

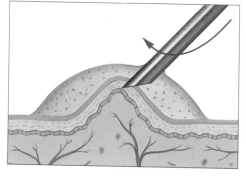

**PRICKING THE SKIN**
*The allergist pricks through the drop into the outer skin and watches for the wheal-and-flare response to appear 10 to 15 minutes later.*

movements of the pendulum he or she makes a diagnosis. Clairvoyant powers are offered as one explanation for the phenomenon. Practitioners of impeccable integrity—many of whom refuse to take payment for this work—have reported excellent results, far better than the 60 percent success rate that would be expected from lucky guesswork. Anecdotal evidence, however, is not the same as a controlled study.

## Pulse rate changes

A modern version of the traditional Chinese auriculocardiac reflex test—in which practitioners look for changes in pulse when a patient is exposed to possible allergens—was devised by the American physician Arthur Coca in the 1940s. An important figure in the early study of allergies and one of the team that proposed the term "atopy" (see page 18), Coca claimed that challenging an allergic patient with a trigger food produced detectable changes in pulse rate. However, pulse changes are held to be unreliable by conventional medical practitioners.

## Cytotoxic test

For a cytotoxic test white blood cells are taken from a blood sample of a patient and incubated with various substances and/or foodstuffs, after which a technician examines the specimens to see what damage has been sustained. The claim is that blood cells from different people will show different patterns of damage to the cells, and substances that cause this damage—said to be cytotoxic—are deemed to be allergenic or toxic for that patient.

This test is believed by some practitioners to be the most convincing one for Type B allergies, but has a high rate of false-positive and false-negative results. There is no proof that it is useful for diagnosing allergies, and several controlled studies have so far proved it ineffective. The test has been severely critized by many medical groups.

## Nutritional tests

Conventional biochemical tests can be used to assess depletion of vitamins and trace-elements in the body that could be caused by allergic illness. Dietary advice and supplements can be prescribed based on the results. Most nutritional tests are carried out on blood samples, but urine and, in some cases, sweat may also be used when

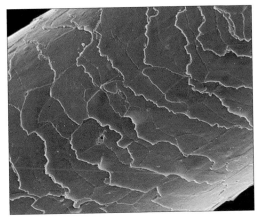

*HAIR TESTING*
*Sufferers of Type B allergies sometimes exhibit high levels of heavy metals, such as mercury, cadmium, or lead, in their hair. Strands of hair are thus used in tests for heavy metals, but the results of such tests for indicating are questionable.*

appropriate. Often the quality and accuracy of these test results may depend largely on the laboratory carrying them out, making them unreliable in general.

## Applied kinesiology

Practitioners of applied kinesiology, also called the muscle weakness test, claim that they can detect changes in muscle strength when a patient holds a glass vial and reacts to a suspect allergen contained in it. The patient is said to be allergic to substances that caused the muscles to go weak. Theories involving bioelectromagnetism have been advanced to explain the phenomenon. In expert hands this method seems to have some success, and the allergens identified often correspond closely to those suggested

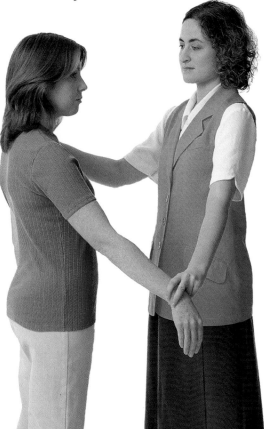

*APPLIED KINESIOLOGY*
*A kinesiologist attempts to detect fluctuations in muscle strength by pushing against or resisting a patient's attempts to move. If a patient grows weaker while holding a certain substance, the kinesiologist diagnoses an allergy to that substance.*

*VEGA TESTING*
*Changes in conductivity at a particular acupressure point when an allergen is inserted there are said to reveal that a patient has an allergy to that substance. Practitioners claim that Vega testing is a noninvasive procedure that gives quick, reliable diagnoses. Rigorous, controlled studies have yet to be done, so it is difficult to assess these claims objectively, and the vega test is not yet approved in North America.*

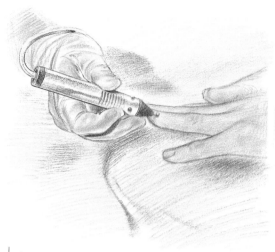

by patients' histories, food challenges, and conventional tests. However, when several different practitioners have been asked to give a diagnosis for the same patient, the results have varied greatly. The indications are that practitioners differ too much in their interpretation of the method and their skills in applying it for this to be a reliable diagnostic tool for allergy.

## IgG ELISA testing

A new and relatively unproven development, IgG ELISA testing potentially offers the same degree of scientific rigor as IgE testing. It looks for the presence of IgG antibodies in the patient's blood. IgG is involved in Type II and III allergies, especially food allergies, where reactions are delayed. So this procedure might extend the range of conventional allergy testing to include a wider variety of allergies.

## Vega testing

According to acupuncturists electrical resistance of the skin varies, particularly around acupuncture points. The Vega test exploits this property by measuring changes in skin conductivity when a vial containing an allergen is inserted into a circuit. If changes occur, the patient is deemed to be allergic.

### HOW EFFECTIVE ARE TESTS?

The fact that there are so many different tests for allergy indicates that none of them is perfect. Even the best tests for allergies have significant error rates and seem to have a limited applicability as well.

RAST testing, basophil degranulation testing, and skin testing have all been assessed for accuracy in hay fever. This is a good condition to use for making compar-

isons because hay fever is usually clear-cut enough to make a diagnosis based solely on the symptoms. All three tests give correct results in about 80 percent of cases, with false-positive and false-negative rates of about 10 percent each. Thus the tests are fairly accurate in the one allergic condition for which tests are not needed.

## Shortfalls

The tests viewed by conventional doctors as the standard ones for allergy—skin scratch, skin prick, and RAST—are useful when it comes to Type I food reactions. In cases of Type B allergies, for which a reliable test is urgently needed, they are virtually useless. The only reliable and reproduceable method of diagnosing Type B allergy that comes up to rigorous scientific criteria is the double-blind challenge (see page 33).

In general, allergists find that intelligent suggestions based on informed guesswork will have roughly a 60 percent success rate. Treatments based on test diagnoses yield a similar result. To properly assess which test is best, more controlled trials are needed. As a result, many allergists rely on a process of trial and error, which remains the best option available so far.

### WHAT IF TESTING IS INCONCLUSIVE?

Allergy testing is never 100 percent reliable. The best figures available indicate a total inaccuracy rate of 25 percent—that is, each diagnosis has at least a 1 in 4 chance of being wrong. Some of the less conventional methods might give better results, but there is no hard proof to back up the claims for them.

Allergists adopt various strategies to cope with this uncertainty. Some choose to ignore it. Patients should be very careful of practitioners who claim to have an infallible test method. Responsible allergists may rely on some guesswork, as explained above, but generally use tests of various types as a starting point for elimination trials.

It should be remembered that all medical treatments are to some extent experiments because a doctor never knows with absolute certainty that a treatment will work in a particular case. A doctor feels that the diagnosis is correct when the patient is cured, and even then he or she cannot be sure. To some degree all medical diagnoses are tentative, and this applies to allergies more than to other conditions.

# CHAPTER 2

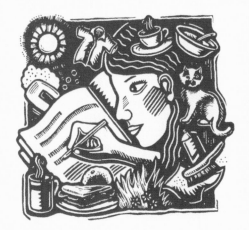

# TREATING ALLERGIES

*Different schools of allergists agree that
the first line of defense against any allergy is
avoidance of the triggers. They also agree that
stress and poor mental health can exacerbate and
perhaps even cause many allergic symptoms, so
comprehensive treatment must involve a mental
perspective. Where experts differ is over the
form that active treatment should take.*

# KEEPING ALLERGIES IN PERSPECTIVE

*The power of the mind to influence health has long fascinated doctors. Allergy research suggests that psychological factors definitely play a role in some allergy problems.*

Almost 60 million people in North American suffer from allergies, and there is a wide range of allergens—allergy-producing substances— that cause allergic symptoms. People can react to an allergen in different ways. The reaction may be an immediate and acute response to an obvious allergen: for example, sneezing after exposure to grass pollen. Or it may be a delayed reaction to a food or something in the environment. The second type is more difficult to spot because the symptoms may be more general, such as a headache in response to a food. The cause of delayed allergy is not always a single food or environmental allergen; it may be a result of many different factors.

### IS IT IN THE MIND?
An allergy specialist uses many different methods to identify the cause of a patient's allergic symptoms. The process involves a careful elimination of other causes that may produce allergy-like symptoms. Anxiety, depression, and stress can produce some of the same physical symptoms as an allergy—including fatigue, headache, backache, and indigestion. An allergist must look at both the patient's physical and psychological history before deciding whether the symptoms are caused by an allergy or a mental problem or a combination of the two. Thrown into the equation is the fact that stress and depression can themselves be caused by allergic reactions, so allergies may be producing other symptoms indirectly.

### The power of the mind
One hundred years ago, the American physician J. N. Mackenzie conducted a well-known experiment in which he provoked

asthma attacks in people allergic to roses by using fake paper roses. In 1987 psychologist Harry Kotses added to these findings, when in a study of 30 normal people at Ohio University, he demonstrated that constriction of the airways (which happens in asthma) could also be provoked in normal individuals in response to suggestion.

In 1986 research from Hamburg confirmed the connection between a person's psychological state and physical condition. Results from 44 asthma sufferers revealed that stress was capable of causing an asthma attack identical to one brought on by allergy, regardless of the severity of the subjects' actual allergies. It appears that, in some cases at least, the physical symptoms of allergy can be produced through psychological pressure.

The picture can be even more complicated by the fact that some people with allergies appear to have an increased emotional sensitivity—that is, they are more susceptible to anxiety or depression. Patients who are anxious or depressed are less likely to take their allergy medication regularly, with the result that their symptoms may worsen. In these cases the correlation between psychological problems and allergic conditions is confusing because it is not clear just how much one is influencing the other.

### How can allergic and psychological causes be differentiated?
Because there is some degree of overlap between symptoms caused by allergy and those caused by psychological factors, how do you tell them apart? There is no simple answer. An allergist's diagnosis depends on his or her approach to treatment and a careful interpretation of the patient's medical

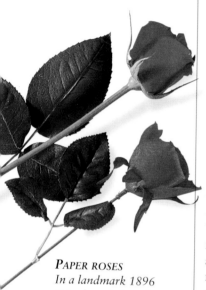

**PAPER ROSES**
*In a landmark 1896 experiment, American physician J. N. Mackenzie discovered that simply the sight of fake roses was enough to trigger an apparent allergic response in some asthma sufferers.*

history. Allergists usually wait until they see the results of treatment before they decide about the main cause of symptoms, but either way, the fact that symptoms are linked with stress does not necessarily exclude an allergic cause.

### STRESS AND ALLERGY

Your emotional state or response to stress can modify your ability to cope with infection, cancer, allergens, and autoimmune diseases. The study of how this happens is a rapidly developing research field called neuroimmunology. Several studies have shown that stress can change both the production of antibodies and the function of white cells, usually resulting in suppression of the immune system. Paradoxically this may actually worsen allergic reactions.

Examples of acute allergic symptoms resulting from stress are "World cup" and "earthquake" urticaria, in which the stress induced by these events has led to outbreaks of allergic skin reactions. In fact, research from Japan has suggested that all chronic urticaria involves a combination of physical and psychological causes. This is not to say that stress alone can cause symptoms. This may be the case in some instances, but in others stress will cause symptoms only if an allergy already exists.

The other side of the coin is that allergic conditions can cause stress. For example, a person dealing with hay fevver while trying to teach a class may find that what is normally pleasurable work is now painful because of the stress of coping with the symptoms.

## Minimizing the effects of stress

It is your own response to stress that determines the effect that it has on your health. When dealt with properly, stress can be beneficial and energizing rather than harmful. There are practical steps you can take when dealing with stress: first, identify situations that you find particularly stressful; second, notice how these make you feel; and third, put into action an immediate stress intervention program (see page 51).

Research has shown that people who are extroverted or exceptionally humorous, creative, or strong-willed, are more likely to have a strong immune system because they tend to deal positively with stress. Sleeping well can also reduce stress levels and enhance the immune system.

## What stress management can achieve

Some asthma sufferers can be significantly helped by psychological therapies. Doctors in Boston discovered that stress management programs helped children with asthma carry out daily activities more easily and with fewer breathing difficulties than those in a control group who had not undergone the programs.

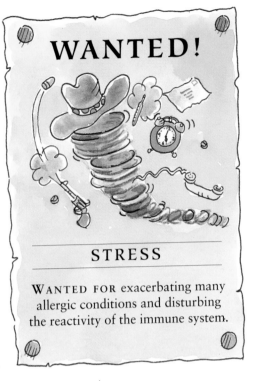

**WANTED!**

STRESS

**WANTED FOR** exacerbating many allergic conditions and disturbing the reactivity of the immune system.

---

## STRESS AND THE IMMUNE SYSTEM

Stress interacts with the immune system in a complex fashion. When under stress the brain triggers the release of hormones from such production centers as the hypothalamus, and chemical messengers from the nerves. These act in concert to affect the cells of the immune system, increasing both the likelihood of initial sensitization—developing an allergy in the first place—and the likelihood of subsequent reactions, and increasing the severity of reactions. These reactions can then feed back, causing more stress by producing allergic reactions and acting directly on the brain to increase arousal and neural activity.

| Stress | → | Hormone production is altered and chemical messengers produced by the nerves are changed. | → | These changes affect the cells of the immune system. | → | Likelihood of initial sensitization increases; the threshold for provoking an allergic reaction is lowered and the severity of the reaction is increased. |

# HOW DOCTORS MANAGE ALLERGIES

*The first step in the conventional treatment of allergies is avoidance of the triggers. When this is not possible, doctors may then prescribe drugs, and some may use immunotherapy.*

Avoiding allergens can be achieved in two ways: by changing your habits to avoid the allergens and by altering your environment to remove them. Evidence suggests that exposure to allergens very early in life may be the number one way in which allergies develop. This means that the best time to start preventing allergies is during pregnancy and the first year of a child's life. This is especially true when one or both parents have allergies, because allergies are to some degree hereditary, and the children in such a family will be at greater risk for developing them.

## Reducing early exposure

A number of findings provide valuable direction for parents looking to safeguard their children against allergies. Preliminary research suggests that avoiding potentially reactive foods (foods that the parents themselves are allergic to) may be important, even during the first half of pregnancy. The period of particular susceptibility to sensitization is thought to be relatively short—lasting up to six months after birth. Studies have shown that infants who are at risk for developing allergies because their parents have them develop less eczema and fewer food allergies if their mothers avoid allergenic foods during late pregnancy and while breastfeeding. Some protein from substances ingested by the mother is secreted unchanged in breast milk and this could sensitize the child to that

allergen. Avoiding the most common allergens (cow's milk, fish, nuts, wheat, and citrus fruits) until 12 months of age can reduce the incidence of allergies among infants at risk. In one study at St. Mary's Hospital on the Isle of Wight, 40 percent of the at-risk infants observed who were not on a special diet developed allergies, compared with only 13 percent of those who avoided the common allergens. Exposure to pets (especially cats) during a child's first year of life also appears to be an important factor in the development of hypersensitivity. Parental smoking has been shown to have a profound effect as well on the prevalence of asthma and other allergic reactions in children.

### AVOIDING ENVIRONMENTAL TRIGGERS

Environmental allergies are caused by substances found in the air or immediate environment and can be either seasonal, such as hay fever, or perennial (continuing throughout the year), such as asthma. Identification is the first vital step in avoidance, and noting exactly when and where symptoms develop can help pinpoint the triggers.

If, for instance, the allergy is seasonal, it is most likely caused by pollens or seasonal mold spores. Avoiding mold and pollens is difficult, although hay fever sufferers can stay indoors more and away from fields at the height of the season.

If symptoms improve or worsen depending on where you are, you should suspect either indoor or outdoor pollutants. Sulfur dioxide, nitrogen dioxide, and ozone from vehicle or industrial exhausts are likely outdoor culprits. Within the home and office cigarette smoke, dust mites, and perfumed products are common triggers.

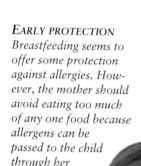

*EARLY PROTECTION*
*Breastfeeding seems to offer some protection against allergies. However, the mother should avoid eating too much of any one food because allergens can be passed to the child through her breast milk.*

## Dust mites and pets

The house dust mite is the most common trigger of asthma and rhinitis, while reactions to pet dander (flakes of skin), hair, saliva, and urine are among the most common allergies suffered today. Preventive measures like using vacuum cleaners with special filters and specially designed mattress covers, washing bedding regularly in hot water (at least 54°C or 130°F), steam-cleaning carpets, and using air filters can all help (see pages 64–68).

### AVOIDING FOOD TRIGGERS

Food reactions can be either immediate or delayed. Immediate reactions trigger symptoms such as itching and swelling around the mouth within minutes of contact. The only proven treatment is strict avoidance of the offending food. Some allergies, in particular to peanuts, can cause anaphylactic shock (see pages 127–128); sufferers should always carry adrenaline in case of exposure.

With a hidden food allergy the body does not react immediately or obviously to the allergen. Common symptoms include irritable bowel syndrome, fatigue, and migraine headache. Hidden food allergies are also treated by avoiding the offending foods, although identifying the triggers can be difficult. A diet-and-symptom diary can help provide some indications (see page 44). Unfortunately, symptoms of hidden food allergy are rarely caused solely by a reaction to one food, and avoidance of a single food may not solve the problem.

## Identifying the culprits

Some conditions are associated mainly with a particular food, for instance, wheat with irritable bowel syndrome. Avoiding these foods for two weeks may help with identification, but this approach succeeds in only a few cases. Constant craving for a certain food, often a sign of addiction, may also indicate an allergy, but a definite diagnosis is reached only with an elimination diet.

## The elimination diet

An elimination diet has to be tried for at least one to three weeks to be effective. This means omitting potentially allergenic foods until the body has had a chance to stop reacting to them. The suspect foods are then reintroduced one by one, and sensitivity to a food becomes obvious as symptoms recur.

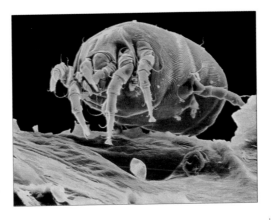

An elimination diet should never be tried during pregnancy or acute viral illness, and prescription medications should be continued throughout the diet, unless your doctor has advised otherwise. Nonessential medications, on the other hand, should be avoided.

After problem foods have been identified they should be avoided. (Some people find that after a period of abstinence they can tolerate the problem foods once again.) It is very important when embarking on an elimination diet to enlist the help of a clinical dietitian. Excluding foods can result in nutrition deficiencies.

### NUTRITION AND ALLERGY

Patients with allergies are often deficient in zinc and magnesium, and some allergists recommend supplements. Zinc deficiency has been associated with impaired immune function, and low magnesium intake may be involved in asthma. These deficiencies are on the increase, possibly due to a widespread change in eating habits. Another dietary factor in asthma may be low levels

*DUST MITES*
*Although impossible to see with the naked eye, these tiny spiderlike creatures can cause or exacerbate asthma attacks and other symptoms. Regular washing of bedding and vacuuming of mattresses, carpets, and upholstery can help lessen the problem. Special coverings for mattresses and filters for vacuum cleaners are available for dealing with dust mites.*

*DIETARY DEFENSE*
*A diet rich in vitamins, minerals, and essential fatty acids can help alleviate the symptoms of allergic attacks. Good sources of these nutrients are vegetables, fruits, fish, and whole grains.*

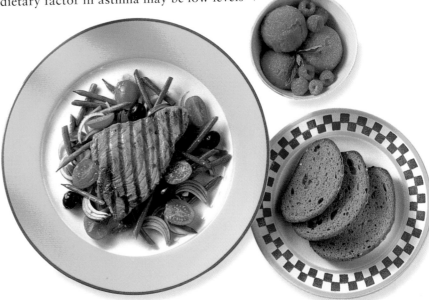

# Identifying Your Allergy with an
# Allergy Diary

*It is easy to lose track of how symptoms change from day to day or even from hour to hour. An allergy diary is a very useful tool for helping you identify which foods or environmental exposures could be causing your symptoms.*

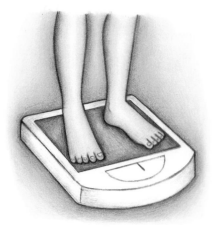

**WEIGHING THE EVIDENCE**
*Record your weight every night after going to the toilet. A sudden gain in weight is a sign of water retention—a common reaction to allergenic foods.*

Allergies can be difficult to identify; keeping an allergy diary is a simple first step in the investigation process that can yield some edifying results. Accuracy is essential to gain a clear picture of what could be triggering symptoms, whether it's a reaction to food or something in the environment.

Simple food allergies may become clear by eliminating suspect foods and recording the results. Hidden food allergies are much harder to detect. It may help to keep a supplementary chart listing all the food you have eaten each day for a week and count how many times a day you ate each food. (This type of allergy is usually to a food that is eaten frequently.) Conclusively relating your symptoms to your diet will be difficult. You may need to do an elimination diet (see page 43).

## ALLERGY CHART

The chart below shows you the kind of information you should record to help expose an allergy and its triggers. Write things down regularly, at least once a day and more often if possible. Remember to note any medications you are taking for your allergies or any other conditions. You could be reacting to one of these drugs.

| | MONDAY | TUESDAY | WEDNESDAY |
|---|---|---|---|
| Symptoms (e.g., headache) | Migraine | Diarrhea, migraine | No symptoms |
| Severity (on a scale of 1–5) | 4 | 3 and 2 | |
| Weight at night | 60 kg 133 lbs | 60.5 kg 134 lbs | 60 kg 133 lbs |
| Medications | Aspirin | Loperamide | None |
| Locations during the day | Home Office | Home Office | Day off (stayed home) |
| Activities | Cooking, cleaning, working at desk | Cooking, working at desk, photocopying | Cooking, gardening |
| Any unusual foods eaten | None | None | Nuts |
| Notes | Migraine came on in evening | Photocopier had a strong smell | Felt better |

## INTERPRETING YOUR CHARTS

After a week or two of keeping your charts, do a series of comparisons to see if there is any pattern to your symptoms and to help you determine any possible triggers. Compare charts from days when you felt ill with days when you felt well, and try to spot the differences in the foods that you ate and the activities you carried out. Certain tasks may provoke an allergic reaction immediately or not until later, even the next day. This may indicate that they bring you into contact with an allergen or that they are a source of stress. Armed with a list of suspects from your allergy diary, you and your doctor will have a much better chance of identifying the substances that are making you ill and avoiding or treating them more successfully.

## COMMON ANTIHISTAMINES

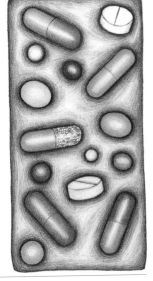

| DRUG | EFFECT |
|---|---|
| Terfenadine | Widely used but can have a rare side effect—heart arrhythmia (irregular beating of the heart). Interaction with certain other drugs increases the chances of this effect, so you should consult a doctor or pharmacist if you are using any other type of medication. |
| Astemizole | Effects take up to 6 hours to develop and last up to 24 hours; traces may stay in the body for up to four weeks after the last dose. The drug's absorption is delayed by food. It can increase the risk of cardiac arrhythmia and cause increased appetite and weight gain. |
| Cetirizine, Loratadine | All three have been shown to be effective without serious problems, as long as patients use the recommended dose. The long-term effects of azelastine and cetirizine are not yet known. Loratadine may be used long-term without ill effects or diminished effectiveness. |
| Triprolidine | Commonly causes drowsiness and thickening of mucus. Should be discontinued at least four days before having an allergy skin test. |

**Warning:** All of the above drugs must be avoided during pregnancy, especially during the first 14 weeks.

of the B vitamins and vitamin C. Large doses of these vitamins can reduce the allergic reaction of asthmatics to airborne allergens, and B vitamins and antioxidants help protect against the effects of stress. While supplements may help (taken under the guidance of a dietitian or doctor), a good diet is also essential.

### CORTICOSTEROIDS
These drugs have an anti-inflammatory and immunosuppressive effect. They work by decreasing the body's production of cytokines—chemical messengers that excite and activate elements of the immune system. They also reduce the release of histamine.

Corticosteroid nasal drops and water-based nasal sprays are effective in controlling the nasal symptoms of hay fever and year-round allergic nasal congestion. They work by reducing inflammation and swelling in the lining of the nose.

Corticosteroids are also important in the control of asthma. Low doses are inhaled as a preventive measure; when taken every day, they can reduce inflammation of the airways and the consequent mucus production. Side effects include hoarseness and a higher risk of fungal throat infections.

Corticosteroids taken by mouth or injection are used to relieve very severe allergy symptoms. Short courses of oral steroids at higher doses may be needed for acute asthma attacks. Prolonged treatment should be avoided, however, because of long-term side effects, which include swelling of the face, osteoporosis, and raised blood pressure.

### BRONCHODILATORS
Bronchodilators help relieve airflow obstruction in asthmatics. There are three types—sympathomimetics, anticholinergics, and xanthines—all of which relax the muscles surrounding the bronchioles and open the airways. The sympathomimetic drugs are used primarily to bring fast relief for an acute attack, while the other two agents are used more often for long-term prevention.

### ANTIHISTAMINES
Many allergy symptoms are caused by the release of histamine, and medications containing antihistamine are a way to relieve them. Antihistamines are effective against sneezing, itching, runny nose, and swelling, but have little effect on nasal blockage.

There are two main groups of antihistamines. The older, classical, ones often cause unwanted side effects, such as drowsiness *continued on page 48*

### WARNING
*Drinking grapefruit juice can be very dangerous, even lethal, for people who are taking certain antihistamines. The reason is that grapefruit juice contains high concentrations of psoralen, a substance that increases the concentration of these drugs in the bloodstream, possibly causing an inadvertent overdose.*

**Cromolyn sodium**
The medication cromolyn sodium—available as an inhalation aerosol, inhalation solution, and nasal solution—can prevent an acute asthma attack if it is used just before exposure to a substance or condition, especially exercise, that is likely to trigger one. It works by inhibiting the release of histamine from mast cells. The inhaled forms of cromolyn are often prescribed for children because they are relatively safe and easy to use. Regular use of cromolyn can help control chronic bronchial asthma, though it should never be used to treat an attack.

# Occupational and Environmental Medicine

*Occupational and environmental medicine (OEM) is a growing practice that includes physicians with many different backgrounds who are concerned with the impact on patients of chemicals and other substances in the home and workplace.*

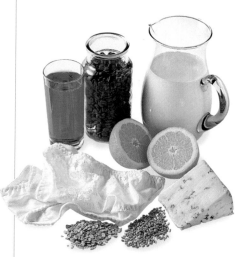

**ENVIRONMENTAL ALLERGENS**
*These include all the substances recognized by allergist/immunologists—house dust mites, pollen, nickel, latex, animal dander, and many foods—in addition to a wide range of environmental substances, particularly in the workplace, that can cause problems.*

## WHY DO WE NEED ENVIRONMENTAL DOCTORS?

The number of people suffering from allergies and diseases caused by contact with toxic chemicals is growing at a rapid rate. Preventing toxic overload is a serious concern for doctors and other health care practitioners today because people in the Western world are exposed to an ever increasing number of pollutants in everything with which they come in contact. Environmental physicians are trained to evaluate patients in terms of their total environment and the impact of that environment on their biochemistry. The aim of these doctors is to pinpoint the principal causes of symptoms and help patients to reduce their toxic and allergic chemical load.

The field of environmental medicine is a broad one that aims to identify and reduce exposure to substances in the environment that cause injury, chronic illness, allergic reactions, and disability. Most of its practitioners have a particular concern with preventing and managing problems that arise as a result of unhealthy surroundings in the workplace or the community and many of them are employed by large companies or government agencies. In addition to treating patients, they may see to it that occupational and environmental risks are reduced or corrected.

(Canada also has occupational hygienists—nonmedical personnel who are trained to anticipate, recognize, evaluate, and control workplace hazards or stresses that may lead to illness.)

## What qualifications and training do OEM practitioners have?

OEM physicians range from general practitioners to otolaryngologists, cardiologists, dermatologists, and other medical specialists who have additional training in such subjects as epidemiology, public health, and toxicology. They generally apply the fundamental principles of prevention and public health to clinical practice.

In the United States these doctors are certified by the American Board of Environmental Medicine or the American Board of Preventive Medicine, and most belong to the American College of Occupational and Environmental Medicine.

In Canada these specialists are certified by the Royal College of Physicians and Surgeons of Canada. Many are members of the Occupational and Environmental Medical Association of Canada.

Another group of environmental doctors—some 400 in the United States and Canada—belong to the American Academy of Environmental Medicine and/or the American Academy of Otolaryngic Allergy, both of which were founded by Theron G. Randolph, the doctor who developed clinical ecology. The followers of Randolph, many of whom continue to call themselves clinical ecologists, believe that numerous people suffer from "multiple chemical sensitivity" ("MCS"), their symptoms brought on by a breakdown of the immune system that is caused by an overload of offending agents. Synthetic chemicals in particular are implicated. MCS is also known by other names, including total allergy syndrome.

Whereas occupational and environmental medicine is a respected practice, clinical ecology remains controversial and has been denounced by some medical groups because many of its tenets and practices are unproven and considered scientifically unsound. However, the lines are becoming more blurred between the two environmental practices.

## Who can benefit from environmental medicine?

Environmental treatment especially benefits people with chronic health problems for which conventional medicine has found no explanation. Type B allergies typically fall into this pattern, with classic symptoms like tiredness, rhinitis, sinusitis, irritable bowel syndrome, asthma, headaches, recurrent rashes, or depression. Many of these patients may be sensitive to one or more environmental allergens but have not been recognized as allergy sufferers.

All of their symptoms need proper medical evaluation, but in many cases the patient has already gone through detailed investigations that have turned up nothing, and their family doctor or a specialist may have attributed the condition to stress or hypochondria.

Patients suffering from occupational asthma, which has become the most prevalent work-related disease in developed countries, can also be helped by occupational medicine. Industries in which a high percentage of workers suffer from this condition include manufacturers of pharmaceuticals, textiles, carpets, detergent, and electronic products. Other workers who are susceptible include animal handlers, seafood processors, hairdressers, and people who install insulation or apply paint, shellac, or lacquer with a sprayer.

## What happens in a session?

A practitioner will take a detailed clinical history, asking about every symptom, its chronology, and the circumstances during or after which it occurred. He or she will also want to know about your general health, family medical history, and lifestyle and what medications or alternative therapies you have tried.

## What tests will be done?

Depending on the circumstances the doctor may do a full clinical examination and blood tests looking at the levels of immunoglobins and white blood cells and possibly for important biochemical information, such as levels of toxins and enzymes or the presence of vitamin deficiencies. Some skin tests may also be done, and if foods or food additives are suspected as triggers, you may be asked to try an elimination diet.

## What treatment will an environmental doctor offer?

The physician may identify some likely environmental culprits and advise you on how to avoid them to prevent further provocation of symptoms. This may mean making some major adjustments around your home or in your diet. Or you may have to request that your employer reduce levels of specific allergens in your work environment or move you to another area.

If avoidance of allergens is not possible, the doctor can prescribe medications that will counteract their effects to some degree.

## WHAT YOU CAN DO AT HOME

Apart from clinic-based tests and immunotherapy injections, most of the steps involved in treating an allergy or other condition triggered by something in your environment must be made by you. There are two stages to this process: identification of the culprit and treatment. While trying to identify an allergen you can help the doctor by keeping a diary of symptoms and when and where they occur, and by observing associations between your health and various environmental factors.

During treatment make sure you follow all the avoidance measures you can manage and all the dietary advice given. You should also take steps to reduce your stress levels. Do more exercise (but discuss what type with the doctor if you have asthma), learn some relaxation techniques, get more sleep, and try some calming measures like meditation.

*PATCH TESTS*
*An OEM allergist may perform some patch tests or demonstrate how they are done, so that you can do them yourself at home.*

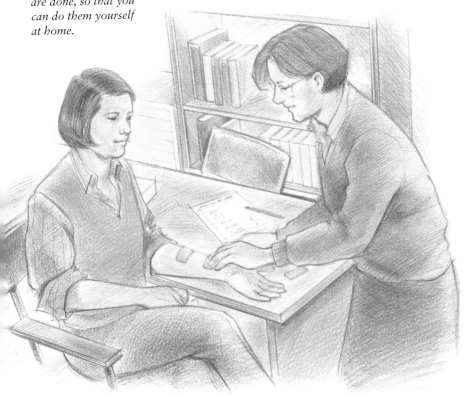

and dry mouth, and cannot be used with other drugs, like sleeping pills and anti-depressants. The newer, selective histamine blockers rarely impair alertness when they are taken at low doses and do not generally have side effects when combined with alcohol or tranquilizers.

## DESENSITIZATION

If an allergen cannot be avoided, there is another form of treatment that offers a potential cure—immunotherapy, or desensitization. This treatment aims to tackle the root cause of an allergy by slowly encouraging the immune system to become less sensitive to the offending allergen, in other words desensitizing it. There are three types of immunotherapy available: incremental dose allergen injection immunotherapy (IIT); neutralization, also known as low-dose immunotherapy (LDI); and enzyme potentiated desensitization (EPD).

### Incremental dose allergen injection immunotherapy (IIT)

This form of immunotherapy involves injecting the patient with doses of an allergen small enough not to produce an immune reaction at first and gradually increasing the amounts until the immune system can handle a normal dose, such as one that would be found in the environment.

IIT has proven effective in the treatment of hay fever, rhinitis, asthma, and allergic reactions to insect venom. However, there is a major drawback, namely that up to 40 percent of those treated will experience unpleasant and sometimes severe side effects, including anaphylaxis (see pages 127–128). The degree of risk depends on the subject's health. Severe asthmatics and other vulnerable patients—people with heart disease, for instance—should avoid such treatment. Until the mid 1980s IIT was popular, but because of the high rate of reactions and even deaths, its use is now limited largely to insect venom allergies.

### Neutralization

Neutralization, (low-dose immunotherapy) involves the use of very low doses of an allergen, which can be self-administered on a regular basis. Patients are tested with mini-injections of the allergen at gradually decreasing concentrations to determine the dose that provokes no localized skin reaction. This is designated the neutralizing dose—the strength of which is just adequate to neutralize the allergic symptoms without causing any harmful side effects. This dose is then given regularly either by injection (two or three times a week) or by drops under the tongue (twice a day). The regimen is continued for months, sometimes even years, until the patient develops tolerance.

Trials of neutralization have shown it to be of benefit for allergic rhinitis, asthma induced by animal dander, and food allergies. In contrast to the higher-dose IIT, this method is reported to give immediate relief of symptoms and it is relatively free from severe or generalized reactions.

The neutralization method has been validated by double-blind randomized trials that show its effectiveness in preventing and relieving symptoms of allergy. It should not be muddled with unproven techniques, such as provocation of symptoms by food extracts, or the use of folk remedies like honey made from flowers containing allergenic pollen.

Note: There is another, similar, form of treatment—also called neutralization—that is controversial and has been largely discredited by scientists. It is employed by clinical ecologists for treating multiple chemical sensitivities, and has been found helpful in only a relatively small percentage of cases.

### Enzyme potentiated desensitization

Enzyme potentiated desensitization (EPD) is based on the discovery that a single low dose of allergen can be made more effective when administered along with an enzyme called beta glucuronidase, which somehow acts to make the allergen appear different to the immune system, so that tolerance develops instead of sensitization and adverse reactions. Clinical trials have shown that one to three doses of EPD per year can successfully prevent hay fever, food allergy, and ulcerative colitis, with few side effects. EPD thus appears to be a powerful and safe method for treating allergies.

There remains skepticism about the effectiveness of the neutralization and EPD methods. A 1992 Royal College of Physicians report in the UK concluded that large-scale trials are still needed. But evidence indicates that these low-dose methods have fewer side effects and are generally safer than IIT.

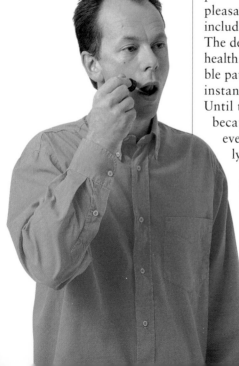

*NEUTRALIZATION*
*Neutralization treatment may involve either injections or the administration of drops placed under the tongue. Once you have been tested to find your therapeutic dose, you will be able to treat yourself at home.*

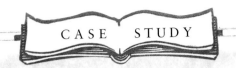
# A Multiple Allergy Sufferer

*There are many allergens in an urban environment that can be inhaled and many potential allergy-causing foods. All of them can cause problems for rhinitis and asthma sufferers. When more than one allergic response is triggered, the effect on the body can be very distressing and the symptoms can interfere with daily activities.*

Robert is a 29-year-old accountant who has suffered from chronic coldlike symptoms since he was a teenager. Recently these symptoms have become worse, and he has experienced a dry throat, headaches, and eye irritation. At work his office is air conditioned; he has a computer on his desk and a photocopier nearby. At home he and his wife have a cat. He eats well and is particularly fond of cheese and yogurt.

Robert's primary care physician tried a number of different decongestants and antihistamines to control the symptoms, but when these produced only a slight improvement, the doctor decided to refer Robert to an allergist to determine the causes.

## WHAT SHOULD ROBERT DO?

Robert should make an appointment with the allergist, who will consider all the details of Robert's medical history. This specialist has the training and experience to pick up on small clues and, once all the evidence has been gathered, will probably suspect that the triggers are in his home and office environment. The allergist will then do skin-prick tests and RAST to determine what Robert is allergic to. He or she will advise him on how to avoid the allergens and will prescribe medication to control the effects of those that cannot be avoided. Although Robert's symptoms do not indicate a food allergy, this avenue will also be explored with an elimination diet.

## Action Plan

**DIET**
*Keep a food diary and, with the doctor's supervision, try an elimination diet.*

**WORK**
*Improve ventilation in the office, opening the windows if possible. Sit away from photocopiers and get a glare-reduction screen for the computer to ease eye strain.*

**LIFESTYLE**
*Thoroughly clean the house, including steam cleaning the carpets and upholstered furniture, and purchase filters to keep the air free of possible allergens.*

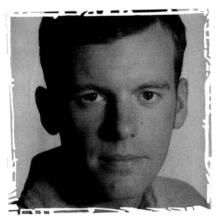

**DIET**
*Milk and other dairy products are among the most common food allergens and intolerances.*

**WORK**
*Air conditioning, computer-screen glare, and photocopier fumes can cause reactions in the eyes and the nasal linings.*

**LIFESTYLE**
*Daily exposure to pets can sensitize people to their allergens or aggravate symptoms for someone who is already sensitized.*

## HOW THINGS TURNED OUT FOR ROBERT

The tests showed that Robert is definitely allergic to cat hair. After giving the cat to his sister and following the allergist's advice on avoiding other allergens, Robert noticed a diminishing of his symptoms. He misses his cat, however, and is undergoing immunotherapy to try to reduce his sensitivity. The elimination diet showed that Robert is intolerant to milk products; he now takes lactase tablets before eating them and has cut back on the quantity.

# ALTERNATIVE TREATMENTS

*Conventional definitions of and treatments for allergies are limited to a narrow range of disorders. As a result, people with chronic symptoms often turn to alternative medicine for help.*

Alternative medicine does not lend itself to being tested in the same way as traditional medicine, because many of the conditions it treats are ill defined, and therapies are often tailored to the individual. This makes it difficult to prove that the treatments are effective. Because of this lack of proof, many doctors are skeptical about the efficacy of many alternative therapies. Nonetheless, patients are attracted by the holistic approach of alternative practices and their gentler, more natural, and less invasive techniques.

### HERBAL REMEDIES

Herbs have long been used for treating allergies. There is little scientific evidence that they work because few clinical trials have been done. However, in 1992 a trial was conducted at Great Ormond Street Hospital in London, using traditional Chinese medicinal plants to treat atopic eczema in 37 children ages 1 to 18. The results showed a decrease in skin inflammation after use of an herbal remedy, with no short-term toxic effects. Another trial applying the same treatment to 40 adults yielded similarly effective results.

Since then, however, concerns have been raised about the toxic effect of the treatments on the liver. Also it is possible that the benefits of these treatments arise from the direct anti-inflammatory effect of some ingredient contained within the herbs, acting like a conventional drug. This suggests that in some ways herbal remedies are similar to conventional drugs, whose side effects are better known and understood. But many trained herbalists maintain that plant medicines have low toxicity and side effects and that they provide more balanced and safer remedies. However, the proper choice of herbs and dosage for an individual should be determined and administered by a specialist. Herbs themselves can cause alergic reactions in individuals with plant sensitivities.

### HOMEOPATHY

Developed by the German physician Samuel Hahnemann in the early 19th century, homeopathy is based on the principle that tiny amounts of a substance that causes the symptoms of a particular illness in a healthy person can be used to treat it in one who is ill. This may sound a little like immunotherapy, but homeopaths use remedies so dilute that a solution may not contain a measurable molecule of the original allergen.

Although scientists do not understand how this approach works, some very careful studies have shown the effectiveness of homeopathy over a placebo (a fake solution with no therapeutic value), even in double-blind conditions (see page 33). A study by Dr. David Reilly at the University of Glasgow showed that a homeopathic remedy containing house dust mite allergen produced significant improvement in 9 out of 11 asthma sufferers. There have been successful trials with hay fever as well.

A homoeopath may treat the hypersensitivity of an allergy and some of the symptoms. To ensure that accurate treatment is received, a trained and qualified homeopath should be consulted. The National Center for Homeopathy in Alexandria, Virginia, has a register of professionally trained American practitioners. In Canada the Canadian Association of Homeopathic Physicians and the Ontario Homeopathic Association provide names of accredited practitioners. Some naturopaths and chiropractors also practice homeopathy.

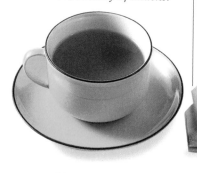

*FENUGREEK TEA*
*As a digestive tonic, a cup of fenugreek tea drunk two to three times a day may help relieve symptoms of irritable bowel syndrome and reduce the frequency and severity of attacks.*

# Beating Stress-Related Asthma with

# Meditation

*It is well known that asthma attacks can be provoked by both acute and chronic stress. Meditation is an effective way to reduce the consequences of stress and calm your breathing, making attacks less likely in the first place.*

To prepare for meditation choose a warm and comfortable environment and make sure that you will not be disturbed for at least half an hour.

## Deep breathing

When you are comfortable, start breathing more deeply than normal into your abdomen and then exhale the breath naturally and slowly. Breathe as slowly and deeply as you can, allowing the breath to push out your stomach as you breathe in. Try not to let your upper chest or abdominal muscles become tense during this exercise. If you simply focus on your breathing, the rest of your body will relax naturally.

## Repeating a mantra

Once you are relaxed you are ready to start meditating. This is often done by mentally repeating a mantra—a specific word—on each exhalation. A monosyllabic word like "peace" may enhance a feeling of relaxation, but you can choose any word you like. The mantra helps to focus the mind. Try to do this exercise for 10 minutes initially. Each time you feel distracted, gently push away thoughts and refocus.

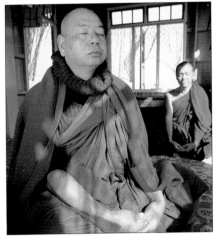

**MEDITATION MASTERS**
*Since the first millennium B.C. followers of the Buddhist faith have used meditation to clear their minds and create a calm emotional state. Meditation has been found to help boost the immune system and stave off allergy attacks.*

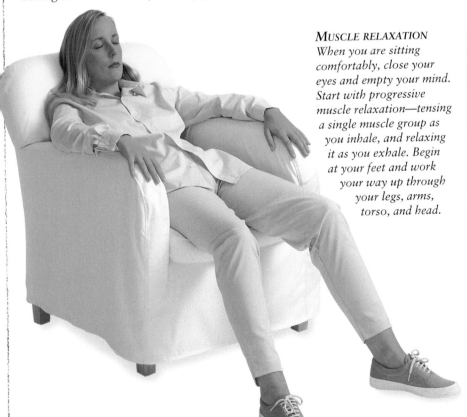

*MUSCLE RELAXATION*
*When you are sitting comfortably, close your eyes and empty your mind. Start with progressive muscle relaxation—tensing a single muscle group as you inhale, and relaxing it as you exhale. Begin at your feet and work your way up through your legs, arms, torso, and head.*

## PRACTICE FOR PERFECTION

A few simple practices can help you maintain your meditation regimen. Each day set aside about 15 minutes at a regular time. Don't allow yourself to be distracted; disconnect the phone and use a quiet, comfortable place. The aim is to minimize your mind's attention on external elements. With practice you should be able to achieve longer meditation periods and greater benefit. If you find it difficult to meditate on your own, consider buying a tape or finding a teacher of meditation. A yoga or t'ai chi teacher could also help you because meditation is part of both disciplines.

## MIND THERAPIES

Just as psychological factors can cause or exacerbate some allergic illnesses, mind therapies can often help to relieve them. The effects of allergies can often be mitigated with practices that reduce stress and enhance the immune system. These therapies take two main forms: relaxation techniques, which include yoga, meditation, massage, and deep-breathing methods, and psychological approaches, which include psychotherapy to overcome mood problems and neuroses, and visualization and positive thinking to improve attitude.

### Meditation

The aim of meditation is to induce a profound state of both physical and mental relaxation. This state is thought to help the body restore its natural healing processes, including those of the immune system. In essence, meditation seeks to activate the body's natural self-regulating functions. Meditation is fairly easy to learn (see page 51), and when practiced regularly, it can help you to become more relaxed at all times. Studies published in the *Journal of Behavioural Medicine* have shown that relaxation can greatly benefit asthma sufferers, and such techniques can help relieve most symptoms of allergic illnesses.

### Creative visualization

Creative visualization involves using mental imagery to improve mood and alleviate symptoms by making positive use of the influence of the mind on the nervous system. The technique has been used successfully to treat both allergic asthma and hay fever.

As soon as symptoms begin, the sufferer clears his or her mind and starts to generate mental images of the different elements of the immune system involved in the allergic reaction, as though directly interacting with and directing them. For instance, lymphocytes and macrophages could be visualized as dwarfing harmless-looking allergens, or the allergens themselves could be imagined as transforming from dangerous red to harmless green. Visualization should be accompanied by constant self-reassurance and assertions that success is possible. As

## STRESS-REDUCING MASSAGE

The massage techniques shown below can both invigorate and relax you and tone the muscles of your face and head. The subsequent feeling of well-being can help to combat feelings of stress and tiredness by stimulating the circulation of blood to the face and head, leaving you refreshed and alert. Facial massage can also help to relieve headaches that might be brought on by food and environmental allergies.

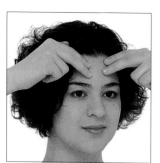

*INVIGORATING STIMULATION*
*Starting with fingers to either side of the bridge of your nose, make small circular movements with the tips, working in a straight line to the top of your head. Continue these movements all over your forehead and scalp.*

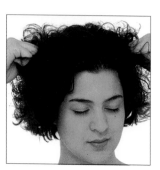

*HAIR PULLS*
*Lay your hands palms down against your scalp and close your hands into fists, gathering up large clumps of hair. Gently but firmly pull your hair until you feel a dragging sensation at the roots. Repeat all over your scalp.*

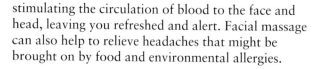

*EAR MASSAGE*
*To complete the massage gently squeeze your earlobes between index fingers and thumbs; rotate the flesh and release. Continue this action around the edges of your ears until you reach the top. Don't pinch or twist too hard. The acupressure points in the ears relate to every part of the body, so you will feel the benefits of ear massage all over.*

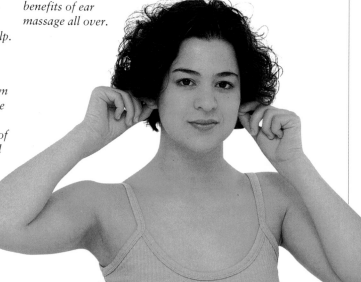

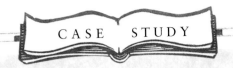
# A Hay Fever Sufferer

*Hay fever sufferers often find that their conventional drug treatments become increasingly ineffective the more they use them. When this is a problem, sufferers must choose whether to keep increasing the dosage of the drug to maintain its effectiveness or turn to alternative therapies, which offer a more natural approach with relatively few side effects.*

Katie is a 25-year-old teacher with a family history of asthma and hay fever. During the past few years she has had regular hay fever starting in May and peaking in late June. She has managed to control the symptoms so far with antihistamines and corticosteroid nasal sprays, but they have become increasingly less effective. Even a newer antihistamine, which is not supposed to cause drowsiness, is making her sleepy. Katie fears that this year's heavy load of exam marking will make things almost intolerable. Her doctor wants to give her a corticosteroid injection but she is not keen on the idea. A good friend told her about the benefits of homeopathic treatment.

## What should Katie do?

Katie should first take some basic avoidance measures, such as staying inside when the pollen count is high and changing her clothes when she comes in from outdoors. To take more positive action, she could consider consulting a medically qualified homeopathic practitioner who is a member of a recognized homeopathic association. In a consultation, the homeopath will listen carefully to Katie's medical history, taking account of such details as the exact timing of her symptoms and her particular physical and emotional reactions at that time. The homeopath will then advise remedies and may suggest ways of dealing with and reducing stress and tension as well.

## Action Plan

**LIFESTYLE**
*Hay fever caused by grass pollens is mostly confined to late spring and summer, so adopt preventive measures during these months.*

**STRESS**
*Consider taking a more holistic approach to treatment, including learning to deal with stress and tension and breaking the vicious cycle that they reinforce.*

**HEALTH**
*Rather than resorting to heavy medication, try a more gentle alternative. Properly prepared homeopathic remedies are safe and free of side effects.*

**HEALTH**
*People vary in terms of how they react to medications. Even drugs that should be relatively free of side effects may cause problems for some.*

**LIFESTYLE**
*Conventional medicines can be more convenient than other preventive measures but may have side effects. Users can also build up tolerance to medications, so that their effects weaken.*

## How things turned out for Katie

Katie found a homeopath who is also a general practitioner. The homeopath tested Katie for common grass pollens to determine her allergens and prescribed three homeopathic treatments. Her symptoms began to improve within days, and she suffered no side effects. In addition she learned a deep-breathing technique to help her relax and deal with stress. When the time to correct exams came around, Katie knew she would be able to cope.

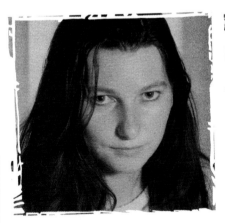

**STRESS**
*Allergies can make a stressful situation worse, whereas increased levels of stress will, in turn, worsen allergies.*

with other mind therapies, the more often creative visualization is practiced, the easier and more effective it becomes.

## Positive thinking

Positive thinking shares many features with visualization but focuses mainly on learning to challenge negative thoughts and stop attributing negative explanations to events. This means taking a positive view of a situation. For instance, instead of assuming the worst when presented with a potentially allergen-rich environment, you can view it as a challenge and a good chance to assert your control over your allergy.

Focus only on your successes—never your past failures—and always talk to yourself in a supportive, noncritical way. Negative thinking creates a vicious circle of worsening symptoms and mood. Positive thinking can break the cycle and reverse the trend. Plan allergy treatments and coping strategies for success and tell yourself that you will achieve your goal. A complete cure is not the aim of this technique; its purpose is to gain control of your allergy.

### HYDROTHERAPY

Two Japanese studies at the Okayama University Medical School in 1992 showed that asthma could be alleviated through hydrotherapy. Why this happens is not clear, although one theory is that the breathing pattern involved in swimming is therapeutic, and the moist, warm air that enters the lungs is soothing. (Asthmatics find dry, cold air harsh and irritating.) In general, water therapies are relaxing, and exercise is therapeutic for many illnesses.

*HYDROTHERAPY*
*One form of hydro-therapy involves swimming in a very warm pool. Studies on the effectiveness of this treatment back up anecdotal evidence that swimming is a good exercise for asthmatics, provided they are not allergic to chlorine.*

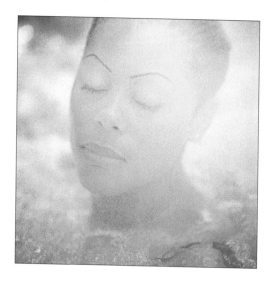

### NATUROPATHY

Naturopaths assess a patient's overall health and well-being and call on many alternative therapies to redress any imbalances or problems identified. Such practitioners place particular emphasis on nutritional therapy to replace any shortage of nutrients and to cleanse the body of toxins.

Deficiencies of some vitamins and minerals have been implicated in allergic conditions (see page 43), so supplements and nutrient-rich foods are obvious treatments. In particular, naturopathy is relevant to the treatment of food allergies and intolerances.

Despite the logical appeal of this therapy, the wealth of anecdotal support for its efficacy, and a number of clinical studies showing it to be effective, nutritional treatment is still considered to be mostly outside the field of conventional medicine.

### ACUPUNCTURE

An ancient Chinese therapy, acupuncture predates recorded Western medicine by at least 2,000 years and is still regularly used in China today. It is based on the theory that *chi*, or energy, flows through the body along energy channels known as meridians. Health problems arise because of blockages or interruptions in the energy flow. By inserting and manipulating needles at special points, chi can be released and used to heal and relieve discomfort.

Traditionally, the acupuncturist selects the points requiring treatment on an individual basis. But in the West a more standardized approach is also used, in which all patients with the same condition have the same points treated. Both methods seem to work well for pain but the Chinese method seems to be better for allergy treatment.

A number of studies—most of which are Chinese—support the effectiveness of acupuncture. A 1993 trial reported in the *Journal of Traditional Chinese Medicine* showed acupuncture to be superior to IIT in the treatment of acute allergic asthma, rhinitis, and chronic urticaria. In Holland about a quarter of general practitioners use acupuncture and believe it to be effective. However, other studies, which have yielded less impressive results, cast doubt on the efficacy of acupuncture. On balance it appears that acupuncture can be effective for asthma, and perhaps rhinitis and urticaria, but not all patients benefit.

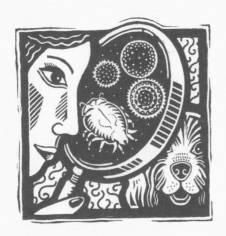

# CHAPTER 3

# AIRBORNE ALLERGENS

*Thousands of airborne, or inhalant, allergens—
tiny particles from chemicals, animals, and
plants—hang suspended in the air all around us
and are taken in with each breath. It may not be
possible to avoid them entirely, but reducing
them is a step toward managing allergies.*

# MODERN LIFE AND POLLUTANTS

*We live in a complex environment that has changed much during the past century. In particular, the air today is filled with an enormous range of chemical and biological particles.*

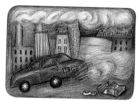

*IN TOWN*
*Asthma does tend to be worse in the polluted air of towns and cities, but the town/country pattern is changing.*

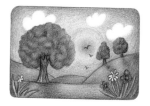

*IN THE COUNTRY*
*There used to be less asthma in rural areas but there are indications that it may be on the increase, for reasons that are not fully understood.*

Rising pollution levels in both the city and countryside are phenomena that concern everyone. Since the Industrial Revolution of the 19th century, factories and chemical and power plants have pumped out smoke and fumes that pose health risks for everyone. In addition, automobile emmissions have become rampant around the world today. Accompanying the rise in pollution has been an explosion in the commonest forms of allergic reaction—asthma and hay fever, also known as allergic rhinitis. These involve the entire respiratory system—mouth, nose, sinuses, throat, and lungs—and cause discomfort, disability, and sometimes even death. Hay fever was unknown until the 19th century, while asthma has become a modern plague in developed countries.

The alarming increases in both asthma and hay fever are linked, and doctors and clean-environment campaigners alike are calling for urgent action to improve air quality and stem the growing tide of respiratory illness. But it seems that outdoor pollution is far from the whole story. The higher incidence of asthma is often blamed on traffic fumes but the condition is sometimes more prevalent in rural areas than in town. On the other hand, hay fever continues to rise in urban areas despite evidence of a fall in the total volume of summer pollens from trees, grasses, and flowers in the cities during the past few decades.

The changing statistics have led experts to look more closely at what is happening inside our homes and offices. Just as outdoor pollution has increased over the past 100 years, so newer fabrics, finishes, and insulating and ventilating systems have led to a radical rise in levels of indoor pollution.

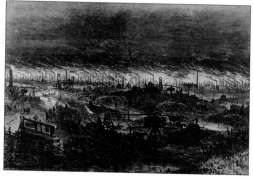

*THE BLACK COUNTRY*
*Industrial pollution was once so heavy in this area of the English Midlands that it was nicknamed the Black Country. Breathing problems and lung disease were common local ailments.*

### INDOOR POLLUTION
There has been an increase in the population of house dust mites within our homes since the 1970s. This decade saw the introduction of heat conservation measures in many buildings as a result of the energy crisis. These measures, including double glazing, caulking, and vapor-barrier insulation have caused a major increase in humidity levels because humidity is no longer dissipated by the drafts that were once characteristic of many houses. Humidity within homes is also increased by the trapped vapors of boiling water, showers, dishwashers, washing machines, rack-dried clothes, humidifiers, and the sweat of humans and pets.

### House dust
The house dust mite needs humidity in order to thrive, and modern houses and living patterns suit it very well. Large amounts of wall-to-wall carpeting and soft furnishings encourage the accumulation of house dust and hence the house dust mite. The

same conditions also encourage the growth of indoor molds, another potent source of airborne allergens.

## Chemicals

There is much evidence that indoor chemical pollution may be the real culprit behind the modern plagues of respiratory allergies. Attention was drawn to the problem as early as 1962 by the American physician and founder of the clinical ecology (environmental medicine) movement, Dr. Theron Randolph. Although he was largely ignored at the time, researchers have now identified a number of sources of indoor chemical pollution that can affect the respiratory system.

Natural gas is used for both heating and cooking in a high proportion of homes in North America. The fuel is less expensive than oil and electricity in many areas and is easy to use but generates nitrogen dioxide when burned. Nitrogen dioxide appears to help sensitize a person to other allergens in the atmosphere (see page 62).

Some recorded nitrogen dioxide concentrations after prolonged cooking sessions in kitchens with gas stoves exceed those found in London's Oxford Street on some of the most highly polluted occasions ever recorded there. Because gas is almost odorless, compared with vehicle exhaust fumes, this major source of pollution has until recently been overlooked. Propane, used in areas where natural gas is not available, produces levels of pollution similar to those of natural gas. Badly installed or maintained central heating boilers can also increase pollution.

Perhaps the next most important indoor pollutant is formaldehyde, and there has been a huge increase in its use in the past few decades. Formaldehyde was used in cavity wall insulation in the 1970s and 1980s, until it was linked to a series of health problems. After a major scandal in the United States, which led to the abandonment of entire housing projects, this use of formaldehyde was stopped. But the chemical is still found in many other elements of the home, including fittings, furnishings, carpets, and ceiling tiles.

Carpets can contain a whole cocktail of chemicals, and there are dozens of other compounds found extensively in houses and offices—cigarette smoke, household cleaning agents, air fresheners, paint fumes, floor polishes, spray perfumes and deodorants,

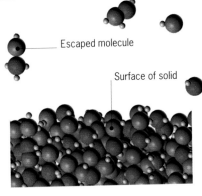

## Outgassing

Researchers believe that the vapors given off by many synthetic materials, in a process known as outgassing, may be responsible for the development of allergic reactions. Normally the molecules in a solid are bonded together and cannot move very far. But at the surface of any solid, especially synthetic fabrics, soft plastics, and glues, a few molecules will escape to exist as vapor.

Escaped molecule

Surface of solid

***ESCAPING MOLECULES***
*In any solid object a few molecules will have enough energy to escape the surface as a gaseous substance.*

and the ink in photocopying machines, for instance. (See page 62 for more details.) All of these pollutants can now build up inside the home because the same lack of ventilation that has increased indoor humidity prevents their escape.

### ALLERGIES AND MODERN LIVING

So why are pollutants important to allergies? There is evidence that inhalation of such chemicals as nitrogen dioxide, formaldehyde, and diesel particles, can affect the immune system in such a way that it is more likely to produce an allergic reaction to substances, like house dust, mold spores, or more benign chemicals, that it should ignore. The immune systems of infants are less able to recognize which substances are harmless and which are dangerous, and so young children are often particularly vulnerable to this kind of interference. If further research confirms this theory, it is possible that air pollution, particularly indoor air pollution, should be considered as one of the major health threats in the developed world. The chemicals to which we are unwittingly exposed could be sensitizing us to the increasingly high levels of biological and chemical particles in the air—both indoors and outside—and setting in motion an escalating vicious circle of allergic reactions.

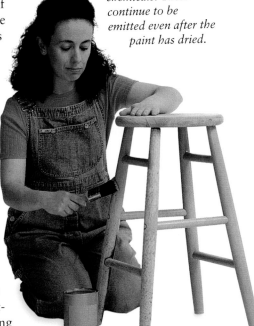

***PAINT HAZARD***
*Common household substances like paint can give off fumes composed of many synthetic chemicals. These continue to be emitted even after the paint has dried.*

# COMMON INHALANT ALLERGENS

*Probably the best-known allergy is hay fever, usually caused by pollen. But pollen is just one of a host of airborne allergens that can cause nasal disturbances and other allergy symptoms.*

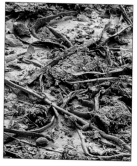

**HOUSE DUST**
*Household dust is a complex mixture of many things, such as grit, skin cells from humans and pets, mold spores, and fragments of insects.*

The entire respiratory system, which includes the lungs, throat, sinuses, and inside of the nose, comes into contact with the air that we breathe and thus with the enormous range of chemicals, vapors, and particles that are found in the atmosphere surrounding us.

### DUST AND THE HOUSE DUST MITE

The melange of ingredients that makes up house dust is one of the leading causes of asthma and the nasal condition known as rhinitis. Among other things, dust contains housedust mite droppings, which can produce a chronic allergic response. This microscopic organism feeds off discarded skin flakes, which we shed constantly. More than 2 million mites lurk in the average double mattress, and it has been calculated that 10 percent of the weight of an average pillow consists of house-dust mites and the dead skin cells that they feed on. Each dust mite produces about 20 fecal pellets a day, and these can cause problems long after the mite dies.

### Ideal mite habitat

Mattresses and pillows are the soft furnishings with which human beings have the most constant and intimate contact. We spend an average of eight hours a day in bed, where we are warm and frequently sweaty. Humidity is vital for the health and survival of dust mites, so pillows, moistened by damp breath and sweat are the ideal places for them to flourish. This is one reason why asthma is often worse at night. Other habitats that suit mites are soft carpets and soft upholstered furnishings.

Mites flourish more in houses with poor ventilation and high humidity—conditions that also encourage the growth of molds. Both can be reduced if the home's ventilation is good enough (see pages 64–67) and the humidity is kept below 50 percent.

### MOLDS

Few people are aware of molds in the air they breathe, but numerically there are about 50 times more mold spores in the atmosphere than grass pollen at the height of the season. Molds need warmth and humidity to survive, and outdoor molds are most prevalent in the summer and autumn. There is a major decrease in the mold count with the onset of the first frost of winter.

Indoor molds are as much a problem as outdoor ones, and in damp houses problems with molds can exist throughout the year. A particular culprit is *Stachybotrys atra,* which can aggravate asthma and cause laryngitis, sore throat, runny nose, nosebleed, itchy eyes, skin irritation, coughing, and fatigue.

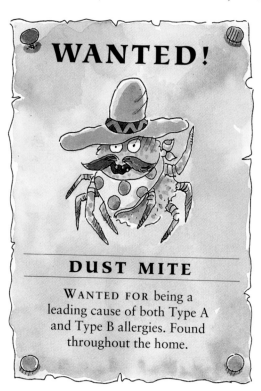

# WANTED!

## DUST MITE

WANTED FOR being a leading cause of both Type A and Type B allergies. Found throughout the home.

### DID YOU KNOW?

Although each house dust mite is only 0.2 millimeter long, it has been estimated that if all the mites in an average double bed were laid out nose to tail, they would stretch the length of five soccer fields.

# ASTHMA

In a study carried out in New York at the [A]
Einstein School of Medicine and published i[n]
*American Journal of Medicine*, asthmatic pa[tients]
were exposed to a range of common odors [under]
controlled conditions. The results were rem[arkably]
consistent. Of the 60 asthmatic patients sur[veyed]

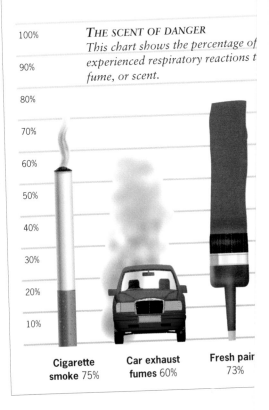

*THE SCENT OF DANGER*
*This chart shows the percentage of [patients]*
*experienced respiratory reactions t[o a smoke,]*
*fume, or scent.*

100%
90%
80%
70%
60%
50%
40%
30%
20%
10%

**Cigarette
smoke 75%**

**Car exhaust
fumes 60%**

**Fresh pai[nt]
73%**

## ASTHMA AND POLLUTION

Between 1980 and 1998 the number of asth[-]
ma sufferers in the United States more than
doubled from 6.7 million to 17.3 million. I[n]
Canada today more than half a million chil[-]
dren under age 19 suffer from asthma. Th[e]
disease accounts for one-quarter of schoo[l]
absenteeism, and some 20 children and 50[0]
adults die from asthma each year.

Outdoor pollutants—in particular dies[el]
and gasoline fumes, ozone, and sulfur dio[x]
ide emissions—can precipitate asthma [in]
sensitive subjects. For instance, the one[-]
unpolluted Isle of Skye in Scotland has [a]
higher rate of asthma than that of man[y]
industrial cities, and the cases of asthma [on]
Skye are concentrated around the port are[a,]
which has a high diesel pollution. Dies[el]
fumes contain millions of tiny particles th[at]
can get deep into the lungs and dama[ge]
them. There are an increasing number [of]
diesel vehicles around, and similar partic[les]

Schools throughout the United States and
Canada have been facing problems with
molds. In fall 1999 a number of portable
classrooms in Montreal were torn down
and scores of others were tested when a
teacher became ill and mold was found
growing on ceilings and walls.

## COCKROACHES

A primary trigger of asthma symptoms is a
protein in the excrement of cockroaches.
These creatures, which have been around
for some 300 million years, are most abun-
dant in urban areas, where they thrive in the
dark recesses of apartment and office buildings. To prevent them from entering your
premises, seal all cracks and crevices, especially in the kitchen and bathrooms. To
treat infestations, use boric acid powder
rather than chemical sprays, which themselves may trigger or aggravate allergies.

## POLLEN

Symptoms of pollen sensitivity are restricted
to the "season" of that pollen. Where pollen
seasons are fairly well delineated, allergists
can use pollen calendars to help them diagnose a patient's particular trigger, and they
may offer desensitization treatments to
reduce the sufferer's response to the trigger.

The most common pollen allergens are the
grasses, which are a primary cause of hay

### ASTHMA ATTACK!

Following a thunderstorm in London
in June 1994 more than 600 people
suffering from asthma filled emergency rooms. Reports in the March
1996 issue of the *British Medical
Journal* suggested that the cause was a
combination of high pollen count and
the conditions of the storm. High
moisture levels could have caused
pollen to rupture, releasing smaller
particles that can be inhaled more
deeply and cause worse reactions.

fever and can also trigger asthma. Pollen
may be implicated in other illnesses as well—
chronic fatigue states, for instance, which
occur only in specific months and can be
provoked by skin tests with summer pollens.

An idea about which specific type of
pollen is involved can be reached by carefully
keeping track of the months in which the
symptoms occur. This is reasonably easy
when the asthma or rhinitis is related entirely to the spring or summer months, but it is
much more difficult if year-round allergens
are operating at the same time.

As a general rule, if a patient has symptoms limited to March, April, and May, the
culprits are usually tree pollen. The most

### WARNING SIGNS OF MOLD ALLERGY

A number of observable
signs indicate that a
person is mold sensitive.
In particular, symptoms
tend to be worse in damp
homes or certain outdoor
situations that include

▶ *Warm, humid, or
rainy conditions,
especially if the sufferer
is near deciduous trees.*

▶ *The period just before
a thunderstorm, when
the rise in humidity
induces molds to release
their spores.*

▶ *Being anywhere near
harvesting, but especially
near combine harvesters,
which throw up huge
clouds of mold spores.*

▶ *The turning over of a
compost heap. This
action releases a huge
cloud of mold spores.*

▶ *The raking of leaves;
rotting leaves are
covered with molds.*

## POLLEN AND THE SEASONS

Flowering plants—which include most deciduous
trees—use pollen to spread their male gametes (the
plant equivalent of sperm). Different plants release
pollen at different times of the year, and many hay
fever sufferers find that their symptoms are worse in,

or entirely restricted to, a few particular months—
namely, those in which their trigger plants are in
season. The exact time depends on where they live:
northerly regions have shorter springs and summers,
while subtropical areas have extended growing seasons.

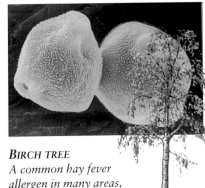

*BIRCH TREE*
*A common hay fever
allergen in many areas,
the birch tree releases its
pollen in the spring.*

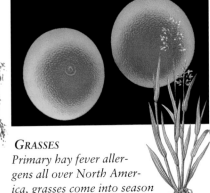

*GRASSES*
*Primary hay fever aller-
gens all over North Amer-
ica, grasses come into season
in May, June, and July.*

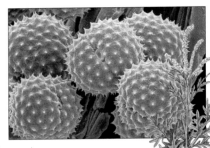

*RAGWEED*
*The most prevalent hay fever
allergen in North America is
ragweed, which is in season
from late summer to first frost.*

## GAS STOVES

Although gas furnaces are vented outside, gas stoves often release fumes directly into the household air. An overhead hood with fan or a downdraft fan between burners can help reduce nitrogen dioxide levels in the kitchen.

### GAS FUMES
*When burned, natural gas releases large quantities of nitrogen dioxide, along with other oxides of nitrogen that may have similar allergy-triggering effects.*

**Toxic molecules**
Paint is usually made from organic compounds derived from crude oil. It often contains potentially allergenic, toxic, or irritant chemicals.

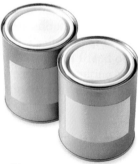

### PAINT
*Substances in paint that are used as solvents can release fumes into the atmosphere.*

Carbon

Oxygen

### ORGANIC SOLVENT
*The fumes from solvents can cause problems for allergy sufferers.*

because of
with the i
inappropri
the body (s

**Nitrogen**
High on th
fere with
dioxide. T
fumes and
an individ
can irritat
upper resp
individual
dust mites
and allergi
pened in
should be
observed
and rats.
human be
  Studies
normal de
enhance
house dus
asthma.
published
showed e
the incid
young ad

**Other g**
A 1995
relations
ness and
dioxide,
compou
ethanol.

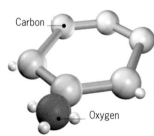

### HYPOALLERGENIC BEDDING
*Pillows and quilts filled with hypoallergenic material (usually polyester) can be encased in mite-proof covers that seal out dust mites but do not trap moisture.*

# PREVENTIVE MEASURES

*Reducing levels of airborne allergens and your exposure to them in your environment are major steps to managing and reducing the symptoms of inhalant allergies.*

The first step toward establishing effective preventive measures for an allergy is to identify what triggers yours, so that you know what you have to avoid. The history and pattern of your symptoms should give some indication of what you are allergic to, but it may require an expert to pin down the exact triggers.

Allergists and some general practitioners stock a range of extracts for carrying out skin tests (see page 36), or they may use a RAST test to confirm their diagnosis (see page 33). You could also see an alternative practitioner, keeping in mind that the reliability of their tests may not have been confirmed by recognized clinical methods.

### INDOOR MEASURES
The preventive measures you can implement indoors apply to most inhalant allergens. Molds and dust mites both thrive in the same conditions. Taking steps to clean up the air in your home and workplace to create a generally hypoallergenic environment and reduce humidity, chemical fumes, and particles will help combat them.

### Reducing dampness
Damp conditions favor both molds and mites, so reducing humidity levels in the environment can greatly benefit allergy sufferers. Make a thorough inspection to find out where water may be leaking in and to identify places where dampness collects or lingers, then take steps to eliminate these problems. Also, increase ventilation so that moisture can escape. Reducing dampness can sometimes involve major alterations, but simple tactics can also make a big difference (see pages 66–67).

Dehumidifiers are very useful for reducing humidity, thus making the environment less attractive to dust mites and mold. These appliances rely on the same technology as refrigerators and work by cooling air. As the air cools, water condenses out of it and is collected in a tank. Air conditioners have much the same effect as dehumidifiers because they dry out the air, but they are generally more expensive.

Relatively low-powered dehumidifiers are sold widely in appliance and hardware stores, but firms that specialize in supplying equipment for allergy sufferers sell more powerful models.

### Controlling dust mites
At an international workshop in 1988 it was suggested that at least a tenfold reduction in exposure to mite allergen was required to improve symptoms in people who are allergic to dust mites. Several approaches are possible. One is to reduce the humidity in your surroundings so that it does not favor mites (see above). You can also attack them directly, remove their allergenic debris, and prevent them from building up in mattresses and bedding.

A study published in the journal *Clinical and Experimental Allergy* in 1995 showed that steam cleaning was very effective at killing mites in carpets. Alternative treat-

**DID YOU KNOW?**
There are more mold spores in the air than any other biological particle. The record in the British Isles is 160,000 mold spores per cubic meter of air. The record pollen count is just 2,800 spores per cubic meter.

ments include chemicals that kill mites—known as acaricides—but these can cause reactions of their own, and studies have shown them to give disappointing results.

Liquid nitrogen is an effective mite treatment; it is extremely cold and freezes the dust mites to death. Liquid nitrogen does not damage carpets or upholstery, but it can be dangerous and must be handled only by trained personnel. The treatment has to be repeated roughly every six months and must be followed by very careful vacuuming.

Tannic acid is another widely available and relatively inexpensive treatment, which makes mite droppings less allergenic rather than killing the mites. It is sprayed onto carpets and upholstery, dries to a fine powder, and is then vacuumed off. One treatment can be effective for up to three months.

Another very effective measure you can take against house dust mites is to enclose both mattresses and pillows in microporous covers. These are made from material that has holes (pores) small enough to prevent dust mites or their droppings from getting in or out, but large enough to let water vapor through. Such covers are available to fit mattresses, pillows, and quilts; sheets, pillow cases, and duvet covers go on top.

Previously, plastic mattress covers were used as antimite measures. They were completely impermeable, however, and a drop in temperature would produce condensation on the inside of the cover. This in turn could lead to the growth of molds, which could then become a major problem if any small holes developed in the cover.

Ideally, you should invest in a new mattress when you get the special cover. If you continue to use an existing mattress, you must vacuum it thoroughly before putting on the cover. Make sure you wash your bedding frequently in very hot water (54°C, or 130°F) to prevent the skin cells that attract dust mites from building up.

## Eliminating molds

Mold spores can make a significant contribution to an allergen load (the total number of triggers that an allergy sufferer's immune system has to deal with) if they are allowed to flourish in the home. It is necessary to reduce overall levels of moisture and scrupulously clean or eliminate likely sites of mold growth, such as showers and tubs, potted plants, and damp firewood.

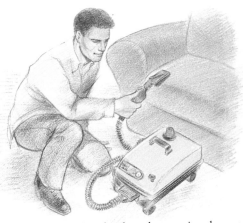

**MITE BLASTER**
*Steam cleaners kill dust mites with superheated steam. You can buy or rent such steam cleaners or hire a professional cleaning company to do the job for you.*

Dusting with a feather duster simply puts more dust and mold spores into the air. To remove dust effectively, use a damp cloth; rinse it under a tap and don't dry it inside the house. Better still, use a vacuum cleaner with a special filter to get rid of dust.

### HYPOALLERGENIC VACUUM CLEANERS

Standard vacuum cleaners are not much use for reducing levels of dust and dust mites. The collecting bags allow microscopic dust mite droppings to escape. These are then expelled from the vacuum cleaner by way of the exhaust and often increase the amount of allergens suspended in the air. Many patients who are allergic to mites report feeling ill after vacuum cleaning. Vacuum cleaners are now available that can eliminate this effect. Most have bags designed to retain the allergenic particles and these are backed up by a special filter that cleans the exhaust air before it leaves the machine. If you can't replace your vacuum cleaner, you may be able to buy special bags or filters to fit your existing one.

### AIR PURIFIERS

There are four main types of air purifiers: ionizers, charcoal (activated carbon) filters, electrostatic air cleaners, and electronic air cleaners. Improving ventilation, particularly in the bedroom, may eliminate the need for an air-cleaning device, but if you believe you can benefit from one, it pays to do a little research because new and improved models are being developed regularly.

**LOW-EMISSION VACUUM CLEANERS**
*Normal vacuums allow tiny particles to slip through the bag, and they remain suspended in the air for up to eight hours. Allergy sufferers can benefit from a cleaner that captures and retains these particles.*

# Hypoallergenic Home

*Keeping your home free of allergens is a difficult task, but there are dozens of ways you can fight dust mites and molds, improve ventilation, keep out dampness, and cope with pets.*

The first line of battle in the war against allergens is at home. Modern housing tends to restrict the circulation of air and may even be geared specifically to prevent air (and therefore heat) from getting in or out. This encourages molds and dust mites by preventing the escape of moisture and also leads to the buildup of fumes and vapors. People with severe, chronic allergy symptoms may be prepared to go to any lengths to improve conditions in their home, but most of the steps outlined here do not involve major modifications. Follow the checklists to make sure that you don't miss anything.

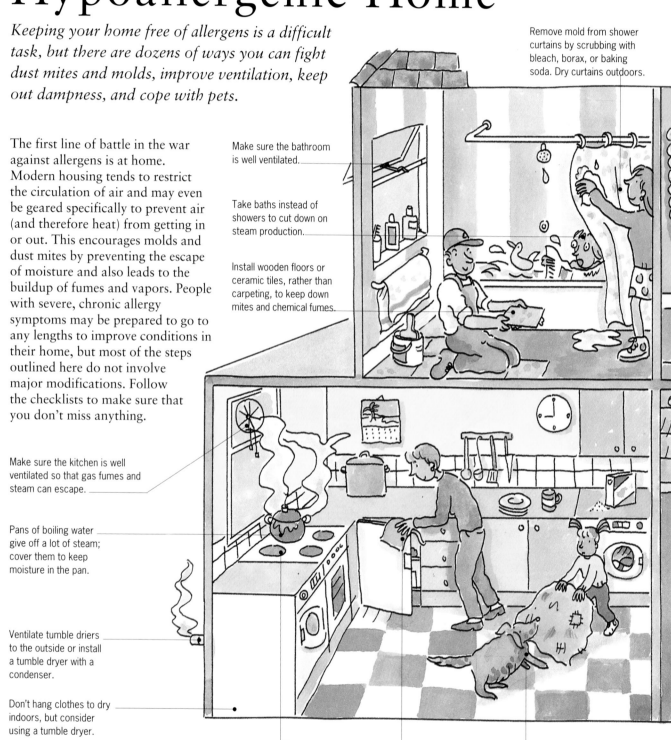

Remove mold from shower curtains by scrubbing with bleach, borax, or baking soda. Dry curtains outdoors.

Make sure the bathroom is well ventilated.

Take baths instead of showers to cut down on steam production.

Install wooden floors or ceramic tiles, rather than carpeting, to keep down mites and chemical fumes.

Make sure the kitchen is well ventilated so that gas fumes and steam can escape.

Pans of boiling water give off a lot of steam; cover them to keep moisture in the pan.

Ventilate tumble driers to the outside or install a tumble dryer with a condenser.

Don't hang clothes to dry indoors, but consider using a tumble dryer.

If possible use an electric stove because gas stoves give off lots of nitrogen dioxide.

The rubber seals around refrigerators are mold hot spots; they should be cleaned regularly.

A pet's blanket or bed cushion can horde a lot of allergenic particles; wash it frequently.

Potted plants are a potent source of mold growth. Put a thick layer of sand over the soil, and water from the bottom.

Keep pets out of bedrooms.

Open the windows to let out fumes and dampness, but keep them closed in pollen season if you suffer from hay fever.

Use an electric blanket to reduce mattress humidity and mite levels.

Use mite-proof coverings for pillows, quilts, and mattresses.

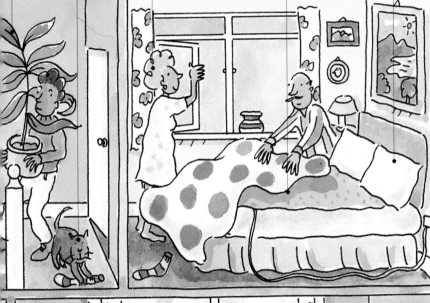

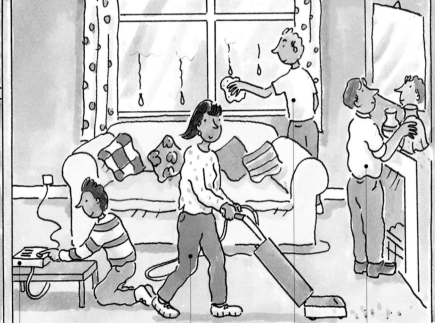

Purify the air with a combined HEPA and activated carbon air filter.

Vacuum often with a cleaner that has a HEPA filter as well as allergen-proof bags.

Mop up any condensation that occurs on windowsills and remove any mold.

For dusting use a damp cloth, rinse it under the faucet, and dry it outside.

## REDUCING DAMPNESS

▶ *Check that the construction material of the house is sound, especially the roof and guttering.*

▶ *In areas with cold winters, install a vapor barrier on the warm side of your home's ventilation. Cover exterior walls with water-repelling material and install drainpipes. Caulk seams around windows and door frames.*

▶ *Seal a clothes-dryer vent with silicone or polyurethane.*

▶ *Insulate any sweating pipes.*

▶ *Use dehumidifiers (see page 65).*

▶ *Make sure that weep gaps on the outside bottom sash of storm windows are not clogged or caulked.*

## CONTROLLING DUST MITES

▶ *Increase ventilation.*

▶ *Washing in hot water (higher than 58°C/135°F) will kill mites.*

▶ *Steam clean carpets to kill mites. Liquid nitrogen treatment by a specialist is an alternative. Tannic acid treats mite droppings.*

## ELIMINATING MOLD

▶ *Make sure no food is allowed to go moldy within the house.*

▶ *Use mold-retarding sprays or solutions such as borax for the bottom of windows, and on the walls surrounding bathtubs and showers.*

## CUTTING DOWN ON CHEMICALS

▶ *Don't use fabric softeners or enzymatic laundry detergents. Avoid strong-smelling cleaning products.*

▶ *Don't use air fresheners or perfumes.*

▶ *Avoid particleboards and synthetic materials.*

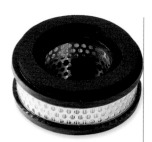

**HEPA** FILTERS
*High efficiency particle
air (HEPA) filters are
made of glass fibers less
than 1 micron thick,
embedded in a matrix
made from larger fibers.*

Ionizers (negative-iron generating) cleaners are portable and relatively inexpensive. Because they are small they are most effective for a single room. Look for one with a cubic-feet-per-minute rating that produces four changes of air per hour. (Note: there has been no convincing proof that ionizers help asthmatics. In fact, the ionization process produces ozone, which itself can trigger an asthma attack.)

Electrostatic air cleaners will remove up to 97 percent of dust, pollen, and animal dander from the air. However, their filters must be replaced every three months.

Electronic filters, which force air through a material that traps airborne contaminants, are effective for most pollutants, including tobacco smoke, bacteria, cooking fumes, dust mite feces, mold, pollen, and animal dander. The greater the surface area of the filter, the better it will perform. The ones of best quality are HEPA filters (see illustration, left), which are more beneficial to asthma and other allergy sufferers than other types. These are now available even as face masks. To clear chemical pollution from the air you also need a good activated-carbon filter, which is usually combined with a HEPA filter; both are available from special suppliers.

## REDUCING INDOOR CHEMICAL POLLUTION

Chemical pollution emanates from materials that are used in erecting buildings and making furnishings, paint and other finishing products, fabrics, and carpeting. It is also emitted from products used for cleaning and air freshening and from the gas or oil used for heating and cooking.

### Gas appliances

Improper installation or operation of a gas stove can result in a buildup of by-products that can cause headaches, dizziness, fatigue, and chronic bronchitis. Gas flames can also produce high levels of humidity and small amounts of nitrogen dioxide; the latter is thought to contribute to asthma in children. (Ironically, the problem may be worse in better-insulated homes that limit air entry.)

You can reduce pollutant levels by making sure the gas burns efficiently (look for steady blue flames) and by keeping the flames from curling up around pots. Your stove should also have a fan vented to the outdoors.

Gas furnaces, water heaters, and clothing dryers that are properly installed and maintained usually cause few problems. However, the filter for a gas heater must be changed regularly to reduce dust particles.

Although the fumes from gas burning fireplaces are drawn up the chimney or out through a wall vent (in the U.S.), some will always escape into the room. You should take steps to improve the ventilation.

If you think any gas appliances are causing you problems, consider installing electric ones. But before embarking on major changes, make sure that gas really is the culprit. Do not use your gas stove or heater for at least 10 days and evaluate your response.

### Formaldehyde

Formaldehyde and other pollutants are given off by many fabrics and carpets, even those made with natural fibers, because of chemicals used in the manufacturing process and to make them stain repellent and wrinkle resistant. Synthetics are the worst offenders. Opening the windows regularly will help dissipate fumes. Consider getting rid of wall-to-wall carpeting because this will help reduce dust mites as well. If possible, buy area rugs that you can wash frequently.

## DEALING WITH PETS

The hair and flakes of saliva and skin shed by pets can be a particular problem for allergy sufferers. Exclude any pet from the bedroom at all times, clean its blanket weekly, and improve ventilation in the house. Desensitization (allergy shots) may also help reduce symptoms.

**WELL GROOMED**
*You can use
a handheld
vacuum
cleaner or a special
attachment for a larger
vacuum to remove
dander and hair
directly from your pet.
Get someone who isn't
allergic to give your pet
a good grooming,
preferably outdoors.*

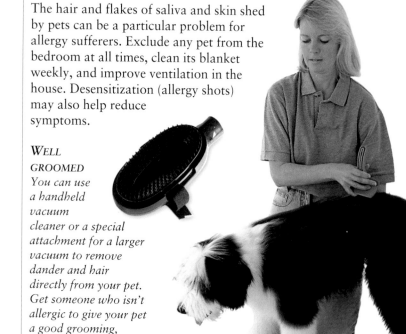

# HAY FEVER AND PERENNIAL RHINITIS

*Allergic rhinitis is one of the most common allergy complaints, causing discomfort and misery to millions. When symptoms are seasonal and pollen is to blame, rhinitis is called hay fever.*

Allergic rhinitis, or hay fever, is an inflammation of the mucous membranes lining the nose and sinuses (see below). The inflammation can be caused by a variety of inhaled vapors and particles. These act as irritants or allergens, triggering the mast cells in the nasal lining to release their cargo of histamine. Inflammation and excessive secretion of mucus result.

Hay fever was virtually unknown until the early 19th century, when London doctor John Bostock described his own symptoms. At first the disease was known as Bostock's catarrh, but the public linked the increasingly common condition with the "effluvium from new hay," and the press coined the term "hay fever." Fever is a rare symptom of the condition, however. It is the respiratory tract that is most affected.

Typical symptoms include sneezing, runny and/or blocked nasal passages, watery, itching eyes, scratchy throat, and a mild cough. The palate of the mouth is frequently itchy as well. Surrounding parts of the upper respiratory tract, like the sinuses and eustachian tubes, can become involved, causing headache or impaired hearing or both.

### TRIGGERS OF RHINITIS

Rhinitis can be divided into two types: perennial, in which the symptoms persist throughout the year, and seasonal (often more severe), in which the symptoms are limited to particular months. The latter is what people usually mean when they say they have hay fever.

Seasonal rhinitis is usually caused by pollen from plants that bloom in either early spring or mid- to late summer, or sometimes by spores from seasonal molds, more common during the fall months. Different types of plants release their pollen at different times (see page 59), so the months when symptoms are worst can give clues as to what sort of plant is responsible.

Mold spores and pollen are by no means the only triggers of rhinitis. House dust mites, pet allergens, and many other airborne allergens can be responsible, particularly for perennial rhinitis, because they are in the environment all year-round.

## Food triggers

Many foods can trigger rhinitis, just as with asthma. Some foods may also cause cross-reactions, in which people who are allergic to a particular plant's pollen may react to foods made from related plants. For instance, someone allergic to mugwort pollen may also react to chamomile tea, made from a plant in the same family. In some cases there is no

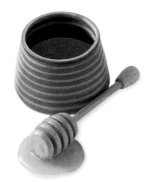

**CROSS-REACTIVE**
*Allergies can be complex, and surprising links can sometimes be found between airborne allergens and food allergens. For instance, ragwort pollen can cross-react with honey.*

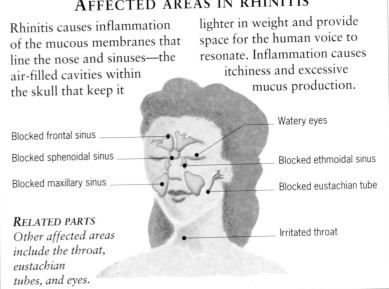

## AFFECTED AREAS IN RHINITIS

Rhinitis causes inflammation of the mucous membranes that line the nose and sinuses—the air-filled cavities within the skull that keep it lighter in weight and provide space for the human voice to resonate. Inflammation causes itchiness and excessive mucus production.

Blocked frontal sinus

Blocked sphenoidal sinus

Blocked maxillary sinus

Watery eyes

Blocked ethmoidal sinus

Blocked eustachian tube

Irritated throat

**RELATED PARTS**
*Other affected areas include the throat, eustachian tubes, and eyes.*

# Avoiding Pollen

*For most people summer is a time to enjoy being outdoors, but for hay fever sufferers it can be a season of misery. Sufferers can follow several strategies to reduce pollen levels in their immediate environment.*

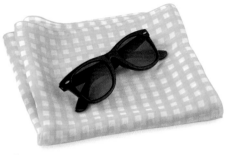

### GLASSES AND SCARVES
*When you go outside during pollen season, some simple precautions can help limit your contact with pollen. Wear sunglasses to help protect your eyes and a hepa mask (see page 68) over your nose and mouth; you can disguise the mask with a scarf wrapped loosely around your neck and lower face. A scarf worn on the head will help keep pollen out of your hair.*

### HOW DOES YOUR GARDEN GROW?
*By minimizing local sources of pollen in your garden and keeping pollen out of the house, you can make an allergen-free oasis for yourself.*

There is not much you can do about the levels of pollen in the atmosphere outside your home, car, or office, but there are a number of steps you can take to minimize the amount of allergen that invades your living and working space. Install air filters and conditioners in your home, office, and car to help keep the air clean.

When you have to go outdoors, avoid walking past fields and grassy areas. Keep an eye on the pollen forecasts and remember that the highest pollen counts occur on dry, windy days and in the early morning and late evening. Plan your journeys accordingly. When you return home, change your clothing and shampoo your hair to get rid of pollen collected outside.

Have someone else mow your lawn on a regular basis to eliminate grass flowers. Also, consider replacing a lawn with gravel, a patio, or a rock garden. This will also reduce the need for pesticides and other chemicals, which can heighten allergic reactions.

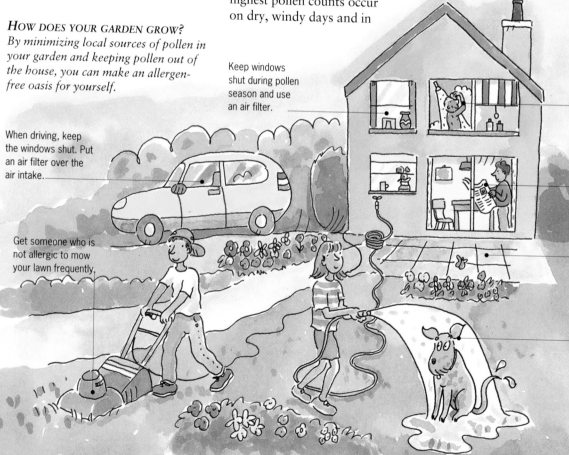

Keep windows shut during pollen season and use an air filter.

When driving, keep the windows shut. Put an air filter over the air intake.

Get someone who is not allergic to mow your lawn frequently.

Rinse or wash your hair to get rid of pollen you have brought in from outside.

Check the pollen forecasts and plan your day accordingly.

A patio or rock garden produces fewer allergens than a lawn.

Pets can bring in lots of pollen on their fur. Keep them out of the house or rinse them off before allowing them to enter.

relation between the different families; for instance, birch pollen sensitivity is linked to allergies to several unrelated foods, including walnuts, apples, carrots, and cherries. These are called coincidental allergies.

### DRUG-FREE REMEDIES

Conventional medications for hay fever and rhinitis have side effects that can create almost as much discomfort as the allergy itself. But there are other ways to relieve the irritating symptoms of rhinitis.

The usual prescription for hay fever is antihistamine, which effectively relieves symptoms but tends to cause drowsiness and dry out the mucous membranes. The mucus may also become thick and clog up the sinuses or respiratory tract, resulting in a dry cough. Nasal decongestants can clear up sinusitis, but after repeated use a rebound effect may occur, causing the congestion to get worse. Oral decongestants can also speed up your metabolism.

## Homeopathy

Homeopathic treatments for hay fever have been proven effective in rigorous trials (see page 50). *Arsenicum album* is good for an itchy, runny nose, sneezing, and watering eyes. *Gelsemium* curbs repetitive sneezing, a blocked or runny nose, and an itchy throat. *Euphrasia* is useful for the relief of red, itchy, watery eyes. Other remedies are often advised to strengthen the immune system.

## Supplements

Vitamin C acts as a natural antihistamine. Increasing your intake during the months leading up to the pollen season may be an effective preventive measure. It is best to get your vitamin C from whole foods, such as fruit, peppers, and broccoli, but supplements may be needed as well, particularly if you are allergic to citrus fruit.

## Folk remedies

Many people take pollen extract supplements a few months before their worst season to desensitize themselves, but there is no scientific evidence that this works, and it may even be dangerous for highly sensitive individuals. The same applies to the folk remedies of taking local bee pollen and honey for the same purpose. No beneficial effect has been shown for them, and there is a slim chance that they might be dangerous for sensitive individuals. Seek professional advice if you are considering trying them.

### Decongestants

Herbs like fenugreek, nettle, anise, and horehound have a natural decongestant action. Half to one teaspoon of licorice tincture, taken in warm water twice daily for five days a week, is also recommended by herbalists, although recent reports indicate that this therapy may carry a risk of water retention (swelling of the ankles, fingers, and undereye area). Inhaling eucalyptus vapors from an essential oil added to boiling water is also an excellent decongestant.

---

## WATER THERAPY

For people who prefer to rely on natural treatments for their hay fever, one simple approach is to use water, plain or salted (½ teaspoon salt per cup of warm water). These treatments can help decongest your blocked nose and sinuses.

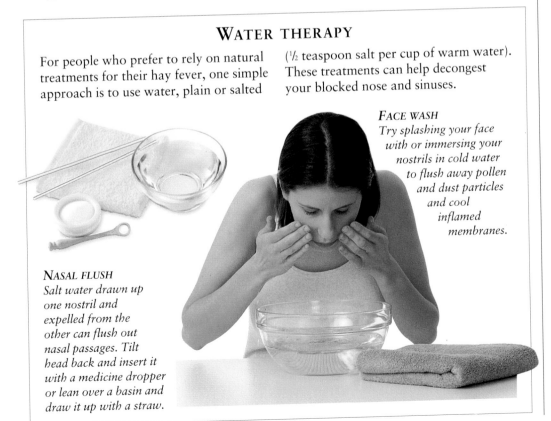

*FACE WASH*
*Try splashing your face with or immersing your nostrils in cold water to flush away pollen and dust particles and cool inflamed membranes.*

*NASAL FLUSH*
*Salt water drawn up one nostril and expelled from the other can flush out nasal passages. Tilt head back and insert it with a medicine dropper or lean over a basin and draw it up with a straw.*

# ASTHMA

*The number of asthma cases is rising rapidly in North America. Between 1980 and 1998 they more than doubled in the United States. In Canada asthma now affects 1 in 20 adults.*

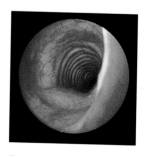

**BRONCHIOLES**
*A view of the inside of a bronchiole shows the rings of smooth muscle that contract during an asthma attack and constrict the airways.*

Asthma, or more precisely, bronchial asthma, is a condition in which the airways become constricted and filled with mucus. The constriction is caused by the contraction of the smooth muscles within the walls of the bronchi and bronchioles, accompanied by increased mucus secretion. These are reactions to irritation of the sensitive lining of the passages by microscopic particles, which provoke an allergic reaction, thus causing the mast cells of the bronchial linings to release histamines and other inflammatory substances.

## SYMPTOMS OF AN ATTACK

Asthma symptoms can range in severity from a slight shortness of breath to tightness of the chest, wheezing, and a dry cough; without treatment they can lead to suffocation and death. The milder symptoms may simply be irritating or uncomfortable, but a severe attack can induce panic and distress. Worsening breathlessness, heavy sweating, and a racing heart lead to low levels of oxygen in the blood, which can cause a bluish color in the face and lips—a condition known as cyanosis.

## TRIGGERS OF ASTHMA ATTACKS

The most common triggers are airborne allergens, including cigarette smoke, but extreme cold or dryness can precipitate an attack in many people, and exercise is a major risk factor (for precautions to limit the effects see page 74). A cold or other respiratory infection can also trigger a flare-up.

Food allergy is also linked to asthma. Milk seems to increase the number and severity of attacks, and such powdery substances as flour, baking powder, and ground pepper can act as irritants. Any food that can trigger an allergic reaction can also cause asthma, but discovering which foods are the culprits can be very difficult.

## TREATMENT FOR ASTHMA

Medication taken through an inhaler or nebulizer is the first line of treatment for asthma. Some is preventive, or prophylactic. They include corticosteroids, cromolyn sodium, and beta-2 agonists; the last is used both to prevent and stop attacks. Others, called bronchodilators, are used once an attack has started to relax and open the airways, allowing more air to flow. These include xanthines, such as theophylline and dyphilline. Steroids are also used to control asthma, but mainly for severe cases because their prolonged use can have major side effects.

Reducing your exposure to triggers and following the strategies on pages 64 through 71 may make you more comfortable on less medication. You can also learn to use a peak-flow meter. This device measures the amount of air that can be exhaled after taking a deep breath and can tell you when an attack is imminent, so you can take prompt action and prevent an emergency.

## AFFECTED AREAS IN ASTHMA

The upper airway leading from the mouth to the lungs is known as the trachea. It branches in the chest to become the bronchi, which branch further to become bronchioles; these in turn lead to the air sacs of the lungs. In an asthmatic attack the bronchioles become inflamed and constricted and produce mucus, causing wheezing and shortness of breath.

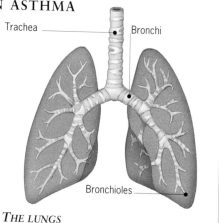

Trachea

Bronchi

Bronchioles

**THE LUNGS**
*The air sacs of the lungs provide a vast surface over which to exchange waste gases for oxygen.*

# Natural Remedies

*Many asthmatics suffer from mild symptoms, which are irritating but not dangerous. To lessen the need for steadily increasing doses of medication, there are some natural alternatives to drugs that can bring relief.*

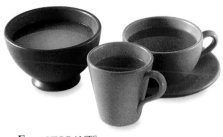

Serious asthma attacks require immediate medical attention, but for milder symptoms—slight wheeziness and shortness of breath—you can try some of these natural remedies.

Warm liquids act as expectorants, making it easier to cough up mucus from the lungs. Half to one cup of a warm beverage like soup, herbal tea, or plain water every half hour or so

relaxes the bronchial muscles. Marsh mallow tea is soothing, and slippery elm, horehound, and seneca root tea have expectorant effects. Passion-flower tea can help soothe asthma provoked by tension or anxiety.

Deep breathing and warm-up routines will also reduce stress-related asthma. Deep breathing utilizes the diaphragm,

***EXPECTORANTS***
*The heat from warm liquids diffuses to the bronchial tubes and dilates blood vessels, relaxing the bronchioles and easing symptoms.*

whereas many asthmatics tend to use the shoulder and chest muscles to breathe, which inflates and deflates only the upper parts of the lungs.

## BREATHING TECHNIQUES

These exercises, developed by the American Lung Association as a preventive measure, can help you learn to breathe more fully and reduce the need for therapy from medications. The routine is effective when practiced for just five minutes every day. All you need is a few moments on your own in a quiet, empty room, preferably one with a comfortable surface on which you can lie down.

**1** *Stand up straight and make all your muscles very tight. Take a deep breath and hold it, tilt your chin toward the ceiling, and hold your arms out straight and stiff. Hold this pose for a few seconds.*

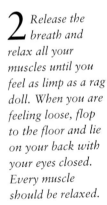

**2** *Release the breath and relax all your muscles until you feel as limp as a rag doll. When you are feeling loose, flop to the floor and lie on your back with your eyes closed. Every muscle should be relaxed.*

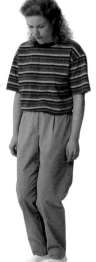

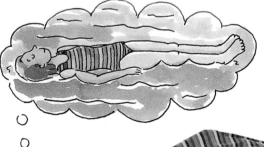

**3** *Imagine you are floating down a river. Concentrate on each muscle, sensing how loose it is. Breathe softly, as if you were asleep, and stay quiet. Whenever you feel an attack coming on, use this sensation of limpness to help you relax.*

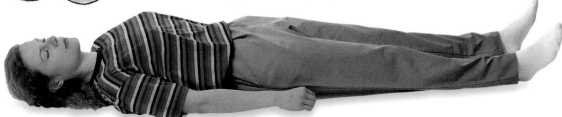

*WATER AEROBICS*
*Exercising in a heated swimming pool, especially indoors, is a good choice for asthmatics because the warmth and the moist air make breathing easier. One caveat is that heavy chlorination can trigger an attack.*

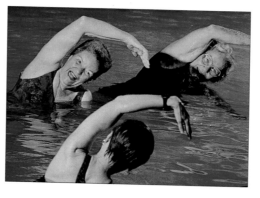

### Preventing exercise-induced asthma

Although exercise can trigger an asthma attack, it can also strengthen the lungs and breathing of asthmatics, so they can get by with less oxygen. It's a good idea, however, to keep an inhaler handy and follow these tips.

Because more asthma attacks occur in the early morning, try to exercise in the afternoon. Choose exercises with built-in rest periods, such as baseball. For jogging or other aerobic activity, slow the pace every few minutes to catch your breath.

Avoid exercising outdoors during cold, dry weather or the pollen season, if these trigger your attacks. Otherwise, wear a mask or scarf to warm and moisten the air you breathe and limit the irritants and allergens. There is some indication that taking vitamin C supplements just before exercise can help relieve wheezing. (A doctor should be consulted for the amount that is effective and safe.) New anti-inflammatory medications—leukotriene receptor antagonists—can also head off problems induced by exercise.

### MAGNESIUM AND ASTHMA

Magnesium deficiency is recognized as an important factor in asthma. This mineral is essential for muscle relaxation; a deficiency makes it harder for muscles, such as those around the bronchi, to relax after they contract. This is what happens during an asthma attack—a process known as bronchospasm.

Two major studies showed that people with a higher consumption of magnesium had only half of the airway hyperreactivity of those with the lowest intake. Asthma sufferers should have the level of magnesium in their red blood cells assessed. Anyone who is deficient should eat more magnesium-rich foods, such as whole-grain cereals, legumes, green vegetables, apricots, and bananas, and perhaps take a supplement on the advice of their doctor, a nutritionist, or a dietitian.

## ASTHMA MEDICATION TABLE

The table below shows the main medications used to control asthma and provide relief during an attack. With inhalers the doses are low and so is the risk of side effects. Some people react to the propellant in inhalants. Powder forms do not have propellants but may contain lactose as filler. Turbohalers contain neither.

| DRUG TYPE | ACTION | POSSIBLE SIDE EFFECTS | EXAMPLES |
|---|---|---|---|
| Preventers | Guard against asthma attacks by making airways less irritable and reducing inflammation. | Throat irritation, coughing, candidiasis (yeast infection). Needs to be taken regularly | beclomethasone, budesonide, fluticasone |
| Nonsteroid preventers | Reduce severity of response to allergens and therefore reduce irritability of the airways. | Negligible | cromolyn sodium, nedocromil |
| Short-acting relievers (inhalers) | Relieve symptoms quickly in the event of an attack. They open up the airways and increase the heartbeat. | Tremors, nervous tension, headache, flushing, dry mouth. Overreliance on these should be avoided. | albuterol (U.S.), salbutamol (Canada) pirbuterol, terbutaline |
| Slow-acting relievers (inhalers); xanthine tablets | Provide longer-lasting relief in the event of an attack by relaxing the muscles around the airways. | Dry mouth, difficulty in passing urine, and constipation (at high doses). Xanthines, which may cause irregular heartbeat and nausea, require close medical supervision. | salmeterol, xanthines such as theophylline and oxtriphylline |
| Oral corticosteroids | Used for control of chronic symptoms. They act to make the airways less irritable. | Husky voice, weight gain, bone thinning, high blood pressure, water retention. May lead to physical dependence. | prednisone |

# CHAPTER 4

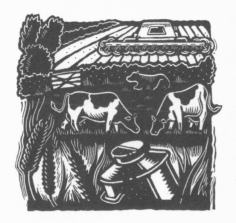

# FOOD ALLERGIES

*Among the least understood allergic reactions are food allergies, which are sometimes confused with intolerances and malabsorption syndromes. Some health care practitioners claim that food allergies underlie a vast range of both acute and chronic disorders and that a significant number of people suffer from either of them to some degree.*

# UNDERSTANDING FOOD ALLERGIES

*There are two types of food allergies: immediate, which produces symptoms within minutes of eating a food, and hidden, in which the symptoms are delayed, thus masking the cause.*

## THE USUAL SUSPECTS

Commonly implicated foods in immediate food allergy include:

▶ *Eggs*

▶ *Cow's milk*

▶ *Tree nuts*

▶ *Peanuts*

▶ *Wheat*

▶ *Soy*

▶ *Shellfish*

▶ *Fish*

▶ *Seeds, for example, sesame*

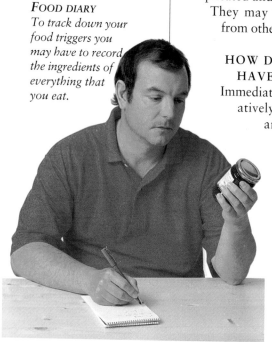

*FOOD DIARY*
*To track down your food triggers you may have to record the ingredients of everything that you eat.*

The two types of food allergy divide along the lines of Type A and B reactions. Immediate ones are Type A; they produce acute allergic symptoms such as swelling, rash, and hives. Conventional allergists typically see these as allergies because they have a recognized immunological mechanism; the symptoms are known to be caused by the action of the IgE antibody. A common example of this sort is peanut allergy. Within a few minutes of eating a peanut, someone who is allergic may experience swollen lips and a rash on various parts of the body.

Hidden food allergies are Type B reactions. Sufferers have delayed onset of a wide variety of symptoms, which may be chronic, and the mechanisms are poorly understood. While immediate food allergies are fairly clear-cut, hidden food reactions are far more complicated and seem to be more common. They may be difficult to distinguish from other, nonallergic reactions.

### HOW DO YOU KNOW IF YOU HAVE A FOOD ALLERGY?

Immediate food allergies cause a relatively small range of conditions and usually involve a fairly limited list of commonly implicated triggers. You should suspect an immediate food allergy if you notice a rapid onset of symptoms after eating a particular food.

Even when dealing with immediate food reactions, however, it may not always be obvious which food is causing your symptoms. A single, minor ingredient may be to blame. If you cannot readily pinpoint the cause, you should keep a food diary. Record all of the food you eat, including snacks. List all the additives (preservatives, colorings, and other enhancers) and all the individual ingredients of recipes, then try to relate your symptoms to a recurring item. A knowledge of hidden food ingredients may help in this detective work (see page 92).

Associations discovered through keeping a food diary are generally the strongest clues to the culprit. RAST (see page 33) or skin-prick tests (see page 36) may help confirm the sensitivity, but these tests are not 100 percent accurate. Evidence gained by observation is usually more reliable than tests. The best route is to avoid the suspect food and see if this prevents the symptoms. If it does, and a subsequent challenge with the food (or eating it by accident) causes reactions, a positive identification is confirmed.

Similar steps may help you to determine whether you have a hidden food allergy. If you have been experiencing a range of vague and/or chronic symptoms, you should have them thoroughly checked out by a doctor. However, if medical investigation does not determine the cause of your symptoms, consider the possibility that they may be caused by a hidden allergy.

### ALLERGIES TO RELATED FOODS

Laboratory tests suggest that closely related foods often share allergens. Blood serum (which contains the telltale IgE antibodies that cause immediate food reactions) from people with an immediate allergy to one food will often show evidence of reaction to closely related foods. Such a cross-reaction occurs, for example, with members of the legume family, particularly between peanuts and soybeans and with tree nuts, such as walnuts, pecans, filberts, and brazils. There is also a cross-reaction sometimes between grains and some fruits and vegetables.

When cross-reactions occur with fruits and vegetables, a link with other forms of allergy is not uncommon—airborne or contact allergies, for instance. A whole range of these cross-reactions has been reported, involving dozens of fruits and vegetables. A a person with an immediate food allergy to members of the botanical nightshade family *(Solanum),* including the potato, tomato, pepper, and eggplant, might, for example, show symptoms of a contact allergy when peeling potatoes.

However, some cross-reactions occur with allergens from plants that are not related. Someone who is allergic to birch pollen, for example, may feel worse after eating certain nuts and fruits. In these cases, allergists assume that the different plants simply happen to share a similar protein or other molecule that acts as an allergen.

### WHY ALLERGIC REACTIONS MAY NOT ALWAYS APPEAR

A variety of factors influence if and when a food will cause an allergic reaction. In some cases, heating a food may weaken or destroy its tendency to cause allergy—its allergenicity. Conversely, a food might produce a reaction only in its cooked form. Other foods become more troublesome after processing—for example, certain fish are more allergenic after canning.

The degree of ripeness of a fruit may affect its allergenicity, as may the effect of processing. In general, ripeness will increase allergenicity and processing will decrease it. Different varieties of the same food can vary in their allergenicity. This effect is especially well documented for potatoes and honey; a sufferer may be allergic to just one variety and will be unaffected by others.

Sometimes a food allergy produces symptoms only through its effect on another allergy. For instance, food allergies may have a priming effect on inhalant allergies. A hidden allergy to cow's milk may cause little or no trouble for most of the year, but during the pollen season the cow's milk could be a priming agent for hay fever. Excluding cow's milk might therefore alleviate the symptoms of hay fever.

A rare but potentially life-threatening reaction to food is anaphylaxis (see pages 127–128). Known food triggers include shellfish, peanuts, tree nuts, pineapple and other tropical fruits, strawberries, some melons, and certain food additives. In a few cases specific food triggers cannot be identified, but there is still a connection with eating. People who have this problem

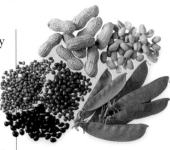

**LEGUMES**
*Peanuts are not actually nuts, but members of the same family as peas and beans—the legumes.*

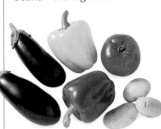

**NIGHTSHADE**
*Eggplants, tomatoes, potatoes, and peppers all belong to this family.*

## FOOD ALLERGY–RELATED CONDITIONS

Immediate food allergy can cause or complicate other allergic conditions, including problems in parts of the body not obviously associated with eating or digestion.

| CONDITION | COMMENTS |
|---|---|
| Asthma | Immediate reactions to foods or food additives may be involved in 5 to 10 percent of asthma attacks. |
| Hives (also called urticaria and nettle rash) | Some 10 to 15 percent of cases may relate to immediate food allergy. |
| Oral allergy (itching and swelling of lips, tongue, and sometimes the throat) | Immediate food allergy is involved in the majority of cases. |
| Laryngeal edema (throat swelling) | Immediate food reactions are often involved. |
| Anaphylaxis (severe allergy symptoms, often with dangerous fall of blood pressure) | Immediate food allergy is a common cause, especially allergy to nuts and peanuts. |
| Eczema | Elimination-diet trials suggest that anyone with persistent atopic eczema has at least a 50 percent chance of having food as a major contributor to the reaction. Although most are examples of hidden food allergies, some immediate food reactions may also be present. |
| Rhinitis (nasal allergy, including hay fever) | Some 30 percent of cases may involve food allergy, although most reactions are hidden rather than immediate. |

# HIDDEN FOOD REACTIONS

*When time elapses between eating a food and the onset of symptoms, this is called a delayed, or hidden, food reaction. It is difficult to pin down the culprit of such a response.*

**Masked allergy**

If the delay between consuming a food and symptoms is long enough and the allergenic food is something common, like milk, reactions may start to overlap and become almost continuous. Some of these allergenic foods may actually be addictive, so that consuming them provides temporary relief from symptoms, and avoiding them can cause a withdrawal effect. This phenomenon is known as masked allergy.

Hidden food reactions are the cause of some of the most intense controversies in the field of allergy research. The contention centers on whether such reactions are true allergic responses or simply types of intolerance.

### HIDDEN FOOD ALLERGY

Some intolerance mechanisms are comparatively well understood (see below), but for the majority of delayed-onset food reactions encountered, the exact mechanism remains unknown. Some medical practitioners regard the symptoms as probably caused by food allergy if they are relieved by avoiding the food and provoked by a subsequent challenge, provided there is no evidence that these other mechanisms are involved.

Most conventional allergists accept allergy as a cause of adverse reactions to foods only when IgE antibodies are involved (Type I allergy). They tend to overlook the symptoms that are caused by Type B allergies or may attribute them to a food intolerance or psychological causes. Because in most cases of hidden food reaction the mechanism is not clearly understood, a definition based on symptoms and response to treatment may make more sense.

### CHARACTERISTIC FEATURES OF HIDDEN FOOD ALLERGY

One of the best ways to define "hidden food allergy" is to explain some of the characteristic features and the problems they pose for sufferers and practitioners alike.

## FOOD INTOLERANCE

Some reactions to foods are neither immediate allergies nor hidden allergies. These are properly termed food intolerance. A number of intolerance mechanisms have been described. The four principal ones are described below, with examples of the foods and substances involved in each condition.

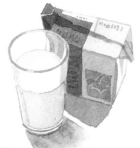

**ENZYME DEFECTS**
*Intolerance can be caused by a defective enzyme in the body; this is the case with lactose intolerance, in which a person cannot break down lactose, a sugar in milk.*

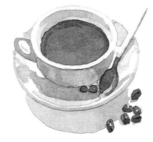

**PHARMACOLOGICAL EFFECT**
*This intolerance is caused by the direct action of a substance in a food, such as caffeine in coffee. The effects in this case are similar to those of a drug.*

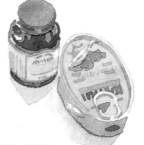

**INTERACTION WITH A DRUG**
*Substances in food may interact adversely with drugs, causing intolerance reactions. For instance amines, found in anchovies, may interact with some antidepressants.*

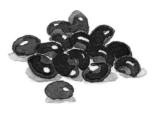

**TOXINS IN FOOD**
*An adverse reaction can result from the toxic effects of a substance in a food. An example is the lectin in kidney beans that have not been properly cooked.*

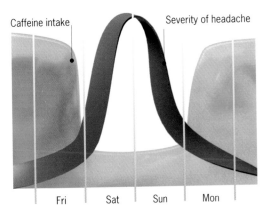

*WEEKEND HEADACHE*
*If caffeine intake drops on the weekend, the withdrawal can cause a "weekend headache," a possible symptom of masked caffeine allergy sometimes experienced by office workers.*

## Multiple symptoms

Whereas immediate food allergy usually produces a limited range of symptoms, in hidden food allergy multiple symptoms are common and, typically, the symptoms will affect a number of organ systems. Also, most sufferers are sensitive to more than one food—usually between three and six but sometimes many more.

## Symptom pattern

Hidden food-allergy symptoms are usually prolonged, but they often fluctuate. The extent to which they fluctuate depends largely on the frequency with which the food is eaten and whether it is eaten in conjunction with other troublesome foods. This variability means that sufferers can almost never deduce the cause of the trouble from the pattern of symptoms.

## Withdrawal effects

Even when a food is causing an allergic reaction, its deliberate or accidental avoidance may precipitate or worsen symptoms. This, of course, makes it harder for sufferers to spot their trigger foods, although an experienced practitioner may look for withdrawal symptoms as a clue. Withdrawal effects do not always occur, however, and the absence of a withdrawal response after avoiding a suspected food is no evidence that the food is not a problem.

## Unmasking

Brief exclusion of a trigger food from the diet, followed by reintroduction, will often result in a swifter and stronger reaction than before. Practitioners may base their diagnoses on this response, which is most reliably produced after one to three weeks of exclusion. Challenging with the food then produces an obvious reaction, effectively unmasking the hidden allergy.

## Timing of symptoms

With a hidden food allergy, worsening of symptoms may show no relationship to when the foods were eaten. After unmasking, certain foods may cause immediate reactions in some patients, whereas in others symptoms may be delayed for as long as two days. Most reactions start between one and four hours after consumption.

## Building tolerance

By completely avoiding a trigger food for weeks or perhaps months, a sufferer may develop some tolerance for it. Maintaining this tolerance will require that the individual remain below the threshold of consumption frequency and quantity that would probably trigger a reaction.

### Theron Randolph (1906–1995)

The American allergist Theron Randolph was an instrumental figure in the early study of hidden food allergies. By the 1940s he had started the clinical ecology movement, identifying and describing hidden food allergies in a significant proportion of his patients. He was also one of the first to describe masked food allergies, particularly to milk, wheat, and caffeine-containing beverages, a pattern he saw among his patients time and again. His work has been expanded to included multiple chemical sensitivies and remains controversial to this day.

## CONDITIONS IN HIDDEN FOOD ALLERGY

Common symptoms of hidden food allergy can involve all areas of the body, from the skin to the cardiovascular system.

Having unrelated symptoms in more than one system can be a telltale clue that hidden food allergy is involved.

| ORGAN SYSTEM | COMMON SYMPTOMS |
| --- | --- |
| Respiratory | Asthma; rhinitis (nasal allergy); otitis media (middle ear infection) |
| Gastrointestinal | Infantile colitis (intestinal disorder causing diarrhea); infantile colic; celiac disease (intolerance to gluten in wheat and other cereals); Crohn's disease (chronic inflammation of the intestinal tract); recurrent abdominal pain (especially in children); diarrhea; constipation; irritable bowel syndrome |
| Skin | Eczema; hives (nettle rash or urticaria); atopic dermatitis (tiny, itchy blisters) |
| Central nervous system | Migraine and other headach; hyperactivity; mood changes |
| Cardiovascular | Palpitations (heart rhythm abnormalities) |
| Musculoskeletal | Joint pain; arthritis; muscle pain |
| Renal tract | Bed-wetting; nephrotic syndrome (kidney dysfunction); nonbacterial cystitis; chronic interstitial cystitis |
| Psychiatric | Somatization disorder (expression of mental and emotional problems as physical disorders); fatigue; hypersomnia (excessive sleeping); insomnia |

# FINDING HELP FOR YOUR FOOD ALLERGY

*Practitioners vary in their approach to the treatment of food allergies. It is important to understand the different approaches in order to find the right one for your condition.*

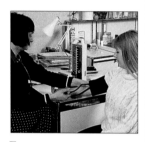

***FIRST STOP***
*Your primary care physician, or general practitioner (GP), should always be the first person you consult concerning unusual or perplexing symptoms. Your GP will be familiar with your history and thus able to see any new symptoms within the context of previous problems.*

Because food allergies are often difficult to identify, health care practitioners can differ widely in acknowledgment of their existence and diagnostic approaches to finding them. The more you understand how food allergies manifest themselves (see page 79) and which foods commonly trigger them (see pages 87–89), the better equipped you will be to find a practitioner who can help you deal with a food allergy.

### THE GENERAL PRACTITIONER

Seeing a general practitioner, or primary care physician, is an important first step for anyone who may be suffering from an allergy because it is essential to have a thorough medical checkup in order to rule out other possible causes of symptoms. On the other hand, a GP's approach to allergies may be limited. A lack of reliable tests for hidden, or delayed, food allergies and the fact that the subject is not covered extensively at most medical schools makes it less likely that a family doctor will consider hidden food allergy when faced with any but the most obvious case. The exception would be a practitioner with a special interest in allergy, who may refer patients to a clinical dietitian. A dietitian can provide the support a family needs because food allergies tend to run in families. In fact, when both parents have allergies there is a better than 60 percent chance that the children will have them.

Although the concept of food allergies is now well acknowledged—they were first reported in Europe in the early 1900s and have been recognized by doctors worldwide since the 1940s—the breadth of related conditions and the range of possible foods involved may be greatly underestimated. There are some physicians who believe that as much as 60 percent of the North American population has symptoms that indicate the presence of a food allergy.

Chronic illness can have a psychological factor, and some doctors will make this diagnosis without investigating further. They may use the term "somatization disorder" to explain patients who exhibit a range of apparently unrelated symptoms for which medical tests show no abnormalities. The term means that an illness is caused by psychological distress manifesting itself through the body. There is no doubt that psychological mechanisms can produce bodily symptoms, and it is known that psychological stress can worsen allergies, but there is also evidence that symptoms attributed to somatization disorder may, in fact, be due to allergic responses.

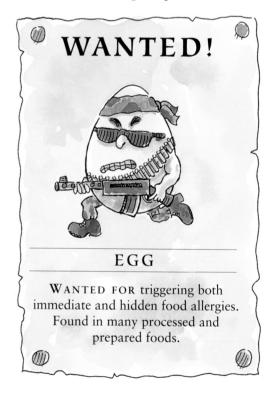

## WANTED!

### EGG

**WANTED FOR** triggering both immediate and hidden food allergies. Found in many processed and prepared foods.

## THE ALLERGIST/IMMUNOLOGIST
A general practitioner who cannot help you with an allergy problem will refer you to an allergy specialist. When making a diagnosis, allergists use skin-prick tests (see page 36) and serological tests such as RAST (see page 33), neither of which can confirm a hidden food allergy. They also challenge with food and/or food additives to confirm immediate allergies. Because they work within the narrow conventional definition of allergies, their interests may extend only as far as straightforward food reactions that have a clear immunological mechanism, in other words, immediate food allergies.

To locate a practioner in the United States call the American Academy of Allergy, Asthma, and Immunology in Milwaukee, Wisconsin. In Canada contact the Canadian Society of Allergy and Clinical Immunology in Otawa, Ontario.

### THE CLINICAL ECOLOGIST
Clinical ecologists are doctors who have adopted a more holistic, symptom-oriented approach to allergies. For diagnoses they use elimination diets and food challenges, as well as the methods of conventional allergists. Most are also concerned about nutrition and may test nutrient levels in blood. For treatment they call on a range of methods, including drugs, diets, supplements, and immunotherapy. They may also consider the role of yeasts and other gut microflora.

Clinical ecologists, who practice mainly in the United States, are considered to be outside the mainstream because they emphasize environmental and nutritional factors. Few of their methods have been validated through double-blind studies, but many patients claim to have been helped by them.

### ALTERNATIVE THERAPISTS
While the severe and life-threatening aspects of immediate food allergies require conventional medical attention, the gentler, less invasive techniques of alternative medicine may be more suitable for treating hidden, or delayed, reactions.

Naturopaths have a particular interest in food allergies. They recognize all four types of allergic reactions (see pages 18–19) in relation to food and advise some of the same diagnostic tests and treatments as a conventional allergist. They categorize food allergies as immediate and cyclic, the latter appearing

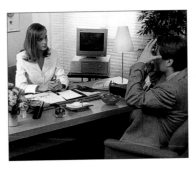
only when a food is eaten frequently. To deal with cyclic allergies, some naturopaths recommend the rotary diversified diet, in which tolerated foods are eaten at regularly spaced intervals to control existing allergies and prevent new ones from forming.

To locate a naturopath, check the yellow pages or get in touch with the American Association of Naturopathic Physicians in Seattle, Washington. In Canada contact the Canadian Naturopathic Association in Etobicoke, Ontario, or the association of naturopathic practitioners for your province.

Unfortunately, there can be pitfalls in some alternative treatments. Many simply do not work, or what works for one person may be ineffective for another. Also, inappropriate or ill-advised dietary treatments may exacerbate conditions or cause problems of their own. Before consulting an alternative practitioner it is always sensible to have a thorough medical examination, to make sure that a serious medical condition is not being overlooked.

### DETECTING YOUR FOOD TRIGGERS
Testing for immediate food allergies should be carried out only in a medical setting because reactions can be severe and life-threatening. However, the essential steps in diagnosing and treating delayed food allergies can be done at home.

The first step is to keep an allergy diary (see page 44). Once suspects have been identified, you can avoid them to see whether your symptoms improve. If this effectively clears your symptoms the next step is to try a food challenge—by reintroducing the suspect

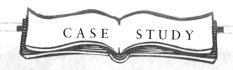

# A Food-Sensitive Sufferer

*Migraine is a debilitating affliction that can last for days and seem to strike without reason. Conventional medications can be expensive and sometimes cause rebound headaches. Certain foods often trigger migraines, and a simple elimination diet can help find the triggers and set you on the path to long-term relief.*

Jenny is 49 and has suffered from frequent migraines since her teens. The attacks have gradually worsened over the years; she has a severe attack every six to eight weeks, in which the pain is usually accompanied by vomiting and difficulty in focusing. Between these bouts she may experience a milder attack, which can last for up to four days. Other troublesome symptoms are swollen ankles (edema) and glands, and puffiness and dark circles under the eyes. She is also overweight, despite generally good eating habits.

Her doctor is treating her with drugs, including an expensive one, for the worst attacks. She has limited her use of the latter to 24 tablets over the previous three months.

## WHAT SHOULD JENNY DO?

Jenny could consider whether foods may be triggering her illness, particularly because of the chronic, drug-resistant nature of her condition. The first thing to do is consult an allergist or dietitian. Following their guidance, she should keep a food diary for a couple of weeks (see page 44) and then start a strict elimination diet along the lines of the Stone Age diet on page 84. If this succeeds in clearing her symptoms, she should continue with food challenges to isolate and identify her potential migraine triggers. Keeping careful records, noting down all the foods she ate, including any additives, and monitoring her symptoms will help her to find the culprits.

(see page 44)

---

### Action Plan

**HEALTH**
*Control the condition through diet and reduce the need for pills.*

**DIET**
*Make a chart of symptom frequency and use it to trace the effects of a strict elimination diet followed by food challenges.*

**EATING HABITS**
*Once challenges have identified the trigger foods, avoid them completely, but compensate for any nutritional deficiencies by creating a balanced diet and taking supplements under the guidance of a dietitian or doctor.*

---

**HEALTH**
*The pain, stress, and other symptoms of migraine can be incapacitating. Drug treatment may become less and less effective and have unpleasant side effects.*

**DIET**
*Frequently eaten foods can cause persistent and debilitating conditions. Migraine is a classic symptom of food sensitivity, as are fluid retention and dark under-eye circles and puffiness.*

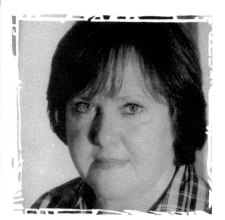

**EATING HABITS**
*Two or more foods could be acting as triggers, the effects of each one masking those of the others.*

## HOW THINGS TURNED OUT FOR JENNY

Jenny had a severe attack at the start of her diet, but then her migraines diminished. After nine days, she started a program of food challenges, and identified four foods that triggered her migraines. They were wheat, chocolate, aged cheeses, and legumes.

By strictly avoiding her triggers, Jenny has not had a headache for three months. She is more relaxed and active, and her other health problems have lessened.

food—to see if it is indeed the trigger. Unfortunately, many hidden food allergies are rarely this clear-cut. Sufferers are usually allergic to between three and six foods, and symptoms will not clear until most or all of them have been excluded. One effective way to do this is to follow the Stone Age diet (see page 84), which, if followed properly, cuts out almost all the most likely food, drink, and additive triggers.

### FOOD CHALLENGES

A clear and convincing improvement in your symptoms after following the Stone Age diet for up to two weeks is the signal to start testing individual foods. Known as food challenging, this is the only sure way to prove that a hidden food allergy is responsible for symptoms. No one who has severe asthma, however, or who has had serious reactions to food in the past, should attempt challenges without medical supervision.

### How to challenge

A food test should be carried out first at breakfast or lunchtime and again in the evening, unless a reaction has already occurred. The food being tested can be eaten either on its own or with permitted or already tested foods. Do not move on to the next food until you are quite sure you have not reacted, because symptoms could be delayed—especially with grains like wheat, corn, and rice—so wait for a day. If you do have a reaction, allow at least 24 hours after your symptoms have substantially subsided before moving on to the next food.

Keep a record chart of your tests. If unsure about a reaction, retest it later, but make sure that you test only foods that you have avoided for at least five days.

### Interpreting your records

Challenging with one food per day may yeild clear-cut results—headache, diarrhea, an itchy nose, and gaining a kilogram (2 pounds) are all telltale symptoms. Even apparently minor complaints, such as poor sleep, irritability, or simply feeling unwell, should be regarded as reactions.

Sometimes the picture is unclear, however. If you felt unwell in the morning but carried on testing and then got worse, was this due to yesterday's food or today's? Both foods must be retested after at least five days of abstinence. If most foods seem to be causing

problems, you may be a slow responder and are not allowing enough time between challenges. Go back on the diet until you feel better and then challenge again more slowly, taking two or three days for each challenge.

### Complications

Remember, you may feel better on an elimination diet simply because you are doing something about your problem (this is called the placebo effect). To be convincing, there should be a clear triggering of symptoms on reintroducing the food or foods. You should also be prepared for much stronger symptoms than before.

If you avoid a trigger food for weeks or months, you may build up some tolerance for it. This can be confusing if you delay testing, but you may train your body to accept a previously allergenic food, within limits.

## TESTING FOODS FOR A CLEAR RESULT

The table below recommends the best forms to use for testing some of the major hidden food allergens. Individual foods should be reintroduced singly and in a simple form. For example, you should not test bread because it contains a number of different ingredients. If you reacted after testing bread, you would not know whether it was yeast, wheat, or another ingredient, like milk, that had caused the reaction.

| FOOD OR DRINK | TEST FORM |
| --- | --- |
| CORN | One fresh or frozen corn on the cob |
| MILK | 8 fluid ounces (1 cup) of whole milk |
| SOY | A glass of sugar-free soy milk |
| EGG | One hard-cooked egg and one that is soft-boiled or poached in plain water |
| YEAST | A quarter teaspoon of fresh baker's yeast mixed into a permitted drink or with a permitted food |
| WHEAT | Two shredded-wheat biscuits softened with water, or a portion of pure wheat pasta cooked in water |
| CHOCOLATE | A piece of dark cooking chocolate (it should be free of milk and milk solids) |
| CHEESE | A number of pieces of different types of very pale Cheddar (test cheese only if there has been no reaction to milk) |
| TEA AND COFFEE | A cup of tea or coffee without milk or sugar |
| CITRUS FRUIT | Wedges of unsweetened orange, grapefruit, or lemon |

# THE STONE AGE DIET

*The Stone Age diet can be a useful elimination diet because it excludes anything that probably was not present in the diets of our Stone Age ancestors more than 10,000 years ago.*

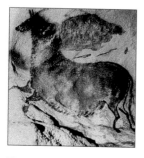

**PREHISTORIC PREY**
*Stone Age art, like this painting from the famous Lascaux Cave in France, dating from 15,000 B.C., illustrates the animals that our ancestors may have hunted.*

One theory about food reactions is that allergies and intolerances result from the consumption of foods with which we are not evolutionarily equipped to deal. The introduction of agriculture and consequent consumption of foods that are now staples, such as rice and wheat, are comparatively modern developments. Agriculture and the domestication of animals did not begin until about 10,000 years ago, and changes have sped up in the past 50 years, with intensive agricultural systems and food manufacture. Our metabolisms and digestive systems, however, have evolved over hundreds of thousands, possibly even millions of years. It may be that the modern diet, rich in foods such as milk and wheat, produces adverse reactions because we are not properly adapted to it.

The Stone Age diet is probably the most comprehensive elimination diet you can follow at home. There are a number of versions; the one given here leaves out cereal grains, sugars, eggs, milk and milk products, chicken, citrus fruits, potatoes, soy products, tomatoes, additives, and a number of other possible hidden food allergens. You can customize the diet to meet particular demands—for instance if you suspect an allergy to fruits. But do not cut out more than one or two extra foods without medical or dietary advice. The table below lists the main foods you can eat.

This diet should be followed long enough to establish that symptoms have cleared up convincingly, usually for at least one week. Only if symptoms have disappeared are foods then reintroduced, one at a time, as

## FOODS IN THE STONE AGE DIET

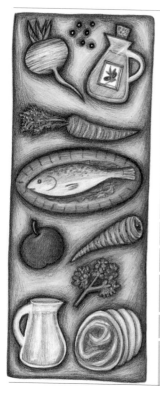

The table below lists the foods allowed on the Stone Age diet; they typify what would have been available to our ancestors who lived in that period. Try to eat organically grown and produced food to avoid possible contamination by pesticides.

| FOOD | COMMENTS |
| --- | --- |
| Fresh or frozen meat | Any kind, including organ meats like liver |
| Fresh or frozen fish | Any kind, but without batter, breadcrumbs, butter, and spices |
| Fresh vegetables | Any kind, except potato, tomato, and soybean (yam or sweet potato can be substituted for potato) |
| Fresh fruit | Any kind, except citrus fruits (orange, lemon, grapefruit, lime, tangerine) |
| Grain substitute | Buckwheat, quinoa (a South American grain) |
| Drinks | Spring water, additive-free juices of allowed fruits, herbal and fruit teas, for example, mint and rosehip |
| Seasoning | Sea salt, black pepper, and herbs |
| Oils | Olive oil, sunflower oil, safflower oil (avoid unidentified vegetable oils) |

food challenges (see page 83), introducing each food for a day only in the first instance. If you suffer from severe asthma, laryngeal edema, or schizophrenia or other mental illness (including severe depression), or if you have ever had a severe reaction to any food, you should not undertake this test without medical supervision.

Keep a chart of your symptoms, starting a week before the diet begins. At the same time, keep your exposure to chemicals, both in the home and in the workplace, to a minimum if possible. Record your most troublesome symptoms on the chart and use a scoring system to rate them.

Weigh yourself on the same scale and at the same time each day—first thing in the morning is best—and record the results. Weight often falls during withdrawal because excess fluid is lost, and it may rise suddenly as a reaction to a food. You may have to weigh yourself at night to detect this effect. If you normally move your bowels less than once a day, take a laxative on the first morning of the diet to help clear out your system.

When an elimination diet produces a strongly positive response, it is not unusual for marked withdrawal symptoms to appear before the symptoms clear. Typically, withdrawal symptoms commence by the end of the first day or the beginning of the second and include headache, aching muscles, and fatigue. Often the last symptoms to clear are weakness and fatigue. In most cases these will have disappeared by the seventh to tenth day of the diet. Take note of any foods you particularly crave or want to avoid, whether or not you experience withdrawal symptoms because craving or aversion can be a clue to the identity of the trigger foods.

If your usual symptoms occur only once every two weeks, or if by the end of a week on the elimination diet you have had no improvement, consider continuing the diet

for another week, especially if you experienced initial withdrawal symptoms but your usual symptoms have not cleared. Work out which two foods you have eaten most frequently on the diet and eliminate these as well for the second week.

If you have been constipated during the diet, elimination of troublesome foods from your system may have been slow. In this case, take a mild laxative on the first morning of the second week.

If your symptoms still do not improve, go back to a normal diet and seek expert help, because it is possible that you are sensitive to one of the foods in the elimination diet.

Remember, clearing symptoms with an elimination diet is no proof of hidden food allergy. Recurrence of symptoms after eating a food is the best proof, and this is where food-challenge testing comes in.

## Keeping well

Long-term proof comes from staying healthy by avoiding food triggers. Both during and after your diet, eat a wide range of foods and try not to eat any one food frequently. Avoid the foods that caused the worst reactions for several months and eat the ones that provoked minor symptoms no more than once a week; this approach may help to increase your tolerance.

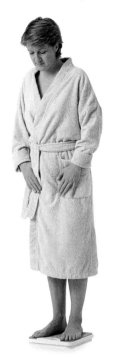

**WEIGHING IN**
*Fluctuations in weight are useful clues. Avoiding your triggers may lead to a rapid weight loss, and positive challenges may cause sudden gains.*

## WATCH POINTS

Additives are not found just in food. Think carefully about everything you normally ingest and try to avoid anything that Stone Age man would not have encountered.

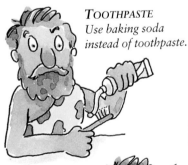

**TOOTHPASTE**
*Use baking soda instead of toothpaste.*

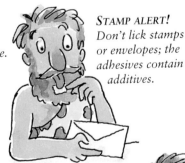

**STAMP ALERT!**
*Don't lick stamps or envelopes; the adhesives contain additives.*

**JUST SAY NO**
*Avoid alcohol and cigarettes; they often cause allergic reactions.*

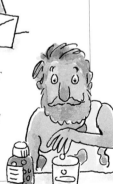

**GRIN AND BEAR IT**
*Medicines contain additives. Stop taking nonessential drugs if your doctor says it's okay.*

# PREVENTING FOOD ALLERGIES

*Little is known for certain about preventing food allergies, but it appears that protection may begin in the womb, and mothers can have some influence on their children's food sensitivities.*

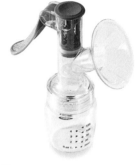

**BREAST PUMP**
*Breast milk is the best infant nutrition. For times when nursing is not convenient, you can use a breast pump to express your milk and store it in a sterilized container in the freezer or refrigerator.*

Genetic factors have a strong influence on the likelihood of developing a food allergy. The prenatal and immediate postnatal environments also seem to play a major role. Another important factor is parents who smoke.

### AVOIDING EARLY EXPOSURE
Whether you develop a food allergy can depend to some extent on the foods you ate when you were an infant and the foods your mother ate while carrying and breast-feeding you. Feeding babies with breast milk for at least four to six months can confer a degree of protection against the development of allergies in general. However, some things that a mother eats can be transferred to her baby through her breast milk, and even cross the placental barrier during pregnancy. This has led to the suggestion that if mothers avoid the foods to which they are allergic, they may help prevent their children from becoming sensitized. It might even help for mothers who do not have allergies to avoid the main allergy culprits, like peanuts, tree nuts, wheat, seafood, and eggs. Research is under way to test this theory.

The best guidelines at the moment are that the risk of developing food allergy is reduced if the introduction of common food allergens is delayed until after the first year. Mothers who are not breastfeeding should give their infants protein hydrolysate formulas rather than milk or soy-based formulas.

Solid foods should not be given until after six months of age, at which time fruits (but not citrus), vegetables, rice, and meat can be introduced—one at a time, to identify any that cause reactions. After one year of age, milk, wheat, corn, citrus, and soy can be added. Eggs and fish may be fed to a child after two years of age. Peanuts should not be introduced until after age three. (Note: peanut derivatives can be an ingredient in some supplements, nipple-soothing creams, and oils for premature babies' skins.)

### ADDITIVES AND CONTAMINANTS
Food additives and such pollutants as pesticides can also provoke adverse reactions in many individuals. For instance, they trigger asthma in sensitive patients. People who suspect they may be reacting to additives and pesticides should eat fresh food as much as possible and buy organically grown produce.

Infants are particularly at risk for having trouble with additives and contaminants, not just because they may develop allergies but also because these substances can quickly build up to toxic levels in their small systems. It is a good idea for pregnant and nursing mothers to avoid as much as possible any processed foods that are high in additives.

## ENJOY THE RIGHT FOODS

Many children eat lots of sweets and junk food, which expose them to additives.

Parents can present healthy foods in fun ways to encourage children to eat better.

*STARTING GOOD EATING HABITS EARLY*
*To limit your children's exposure to food additives, present them with fresh foods, especially fruits and vegetables. Don't introduce babies to allergenic foods, like wheat, corn, citrus fruits, and soy, until after age one, peanuts until age three.*

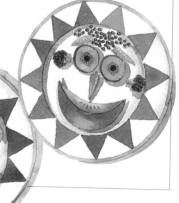

# COMMON FOOD ALLERGENS

*Any food can cause an allergic reaction, but the majority of food allergies involve just a handful of particularly troublesome, commonly eaten foods.*

Why are some common foods particularly troublesome? It is probably *because* they are common that they cause so many problems. The more we are exposed to a food, the more likely we are to develop a sensitivity to it.

Proteins are the parts of foods that most often cause reactions. The most common food allergens—causing up to 90 percent of all allergic reactions—are proteins in cow's milk, eggs, peanuts, wheat, soy, fish, shellfish, and tree nuts.

### MILK AND CHEESE

Milk can cause both immediate and delayed, or hidden, food allergies, and many patients who react to milk suffer from more than one condition or symptom. Milk also causes symptoms of lactose intolerance (see page 97), when an individual lacks a sufficient amount of the enzyme needed to break down lactose, the sugar found in milk; the immune system is not involved in lactose intolerance. The milks from cows, goats, and sheep share several common allergens, and people who cannot tolerate cow's milk may also react to goat's or sheep's milk as well. However, some allergic individuals can tolerate a little evaporated milk. Sufferers should try to avoid milk in all foods, which means reading ingredient lists carefully for such terms as whey and casein.

Cheese can cause nearly all the same problems as cow's milk. In addition, it may contain colorings and nuts or other added foods that cause allergies, and it is generally high in chemicals called amines (for example, tyramine), sensitivity to which can trigger a

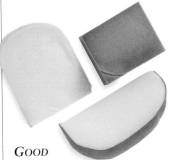

**GOOD CHEESES**
*Gouda and Edam are virtually lactose free and are safe for most people who are lactose intolerant. Norwegian Gjetost, a brown cheese, is made from whey and thus contains no casein, the protein that most milk-sensitive people react to.*

---

## DOES IT MATTER WHAT COWS EAT?

Does the food of a cow affect the response to its milk? In 1925 a German physician reported, "I have… never failed to enquire as to the feeding of the dairy herd, and have had great satisfaction in observing many a seriously sick infant become normal in a short period, if the offending food was eliminated from the diet given to the dairy cattle." An allergy to ragweed pollen, for instance, might be made worse by milk from cows that ate ragweed, but no research has been carried out to confirm this theory.

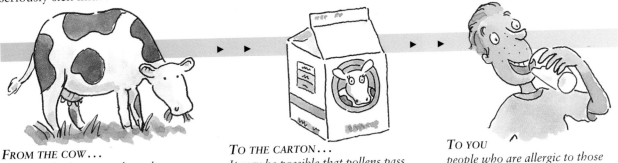

**FROM THE COW…**
*Cows eat both grass and weeds, the pollens of which are frequently associated with hay fever.*

**TO THE CARTON…**
*It may be possible that pollens pass from a cow's digestive system into its milk and cause an allergic reaction in*

**TO YOU**
*people who are allergic to those particular pollens. Research is needed to prove the possibility.*

*Wheat, which is high in gluten, often causes allergies or malabsorption problems. Some other grains also cause difficulties.*

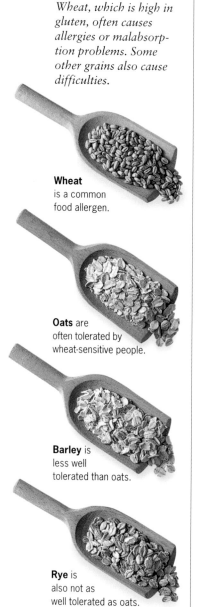

**Wheat**
is a common
food allergen.

**Oats** are
often tolerated by
wheat-sensitive people.

**Barley** is
less well
tolerated than oats.

**Rye** is
also not as
well tolerated as oats.

migraine headache in susceptible individuals. Cheese has lower levels of lactose than milk, however, making it safer for people who are lactose intolerant.

### CHOCOLATE

Chocolate is commonly blamed for triggering migraine. As with cheese, this may be because of its moderately high amine content. However, the same patients may find that foods with a higher amine content do not act as migraine triggers, while other foods with negligible amine content do. Even people who have a major problem with cheese and chocolate may not become migraine free simply by avoiding them because other conditions are involved, too.

### EGGS

Egg, which appears to be a common trigger of food allergy in both children and adults, can cause a range of problems similar to those caused by milk. It may take the form of a rash on the face or an associated swelling of the lips or face. In severe cases there may be wheezing or throat swelling. A delayed reaction to egg is less common, but children with eczema sometimes show a worsening of symptoms that last several days, starting several hours after eating egg.

Sufferers should avoid all foods that contain egg and choose substitutes instead (see page 92), although some people find that they can tolerate eggs that are well cooked.

### WHEAT

Grains of wheat contain a complex of proteins, collectively known as gluten, that give wheat its dough-forming properties. In the 1930s this substance was identified as the cause of celiac disease, a condition in which

a hereditary defect prevents the absorption of gluten and causes such symptoms as abdominal bloating, flatulence, diarrhea, and unexplained weight loss. Untreated, the disease can damage the intestinal lining.

As well as causing celiac disease, wheat is a common food allergen, both direct and hidden, triggering all the typical food allergy symptoms, either alone or in combination with other foods. These more widespread effects may be caused by a part of the grain other than the gluten—the bran for instance. Some patients with irritable bowel syndrome who have been taking extra bran on medical advice appear to be much improved when rice or oat bran is substituted and they remove wheat from their diet.

### Gluten-free foods

Most food labeled gluten free is free from wheat, rye, and barley—the gluten-containing grains. Unfortunately, some packaged foods that claim to be gluten free contain wheat from which the majority of gluten has been removed. Such a product may still be unsuitable for someone with a wheat allergy. Apart from this confusion over labeling it may not always be obvious that a processed food contains wheat. A wheat-intolerant individual should read labels very carefully and consult a dietitian about appropriate substitutes.

### Wheat substitutes

To be safe, wheat-sensitive patients should avoid all cereal grains until they have found which ones are safe for them. Breads made with rice flour or some type of bean flour are usually suitable. Noodles made with rice, buckwheat, Jerusalem artichokes, or soybeans are tolerated, and breakfast cereals are available made with every kind of grain.

### CORN

If wheat is the commonest hidden food allergen, then corn (historically referred to as maize in some places) is the most overlooked. It is present in a wide range of manufactured foods, appearing as corn flour, corn syrup and other corn-derived sweeteners, cornflakes, popcorn, and corn starch. Early investigators of food allergy tended to be concerned mainly with proteins, and the allergenicity of carbohydrates (sugars and starch) was largely overlooked. One problem is that corn has often been used as a

## WHAT'S IN A WHEAT GRAIN?

Different parts of wheat may cause problems for different people. Some patients report that they are more affected by the bran (outer husk) than the kernel (central meat of the grain).

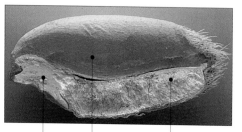

**Embryo**
develops into a
new plant.

**Bran (coat)**
is high in
fiber.

**Endosperm**
is main part
of the kernel.

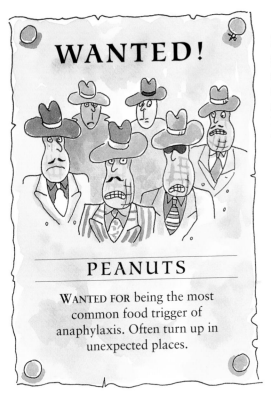

# WANTED!

## PEANUTS

**WANTED FOR** being the most common food trigger of anaphylaxis. Often turn up in unexpected places.

A much wider role for yeast sensitivity has been suggested. It is claimed that some patients with multiple symptoms, including chronic fatigue and exhaustion, headaches, abdominal pain, bloating, and urinary symptoms, improve substantially on a diet low in yeast and sugars, sometimes coupled with a course of antiyeast therapy. This theory is based on anecdotal evidence and remains unproved.

### NUTS

A common trigger for severe food allergy is the peanut, which is actually a legume and a member of the same family as the soybean, another common food allergen. Some individuals are also allergic to tree nuts such as walnuts and filberts. The reasons for this coincidental reactivity are unclear, because many nuts belong to unrelated families.

Peanuts and nuts can cause violent reactions. People who know they are at risk should be very vigilant and carry adrenaline in case of an attack (see page 128). Sensitive persons should also be aware of hidden uses of nuts; they often appear as thickeners and fillings in savory snacks and are common in Oriental, Cajun, and African dishes, sometimes as part of a paste or sauce.

## Why do peanuts cause such severe reactions?

One factor may be that they contain lectins, highly toxic compounds that can have direct effects on mast cells (known as pseudoallergic reactions). Because peanuts are a member of the legume family, and other legumes contain lectins as well, some people who are allergic to peanuts have cross-reactivity with other legumes like soybeans.

substitute for wheat in elimination diets, giving false-negative results. In fact, most manufactured foods prepared for wheat-intolerant patients contain corn.

### SHELLFISH AND FISH

Shellfish and fish are common triggers of immediate food allergies but can cause delayed allergies as well. People's reactions to shellfish vary in severity. One reason is that many shellfish are treated with a preservative called benzoate, to which some people are allergic or intolerant; different batches of shellfish can have different levels of benzoate.

Anyone who has had an adverse reaction to shellfish should be very careful about eating them again and be alert for dishes that might contain them, such as paella and jambalaya. Shellfish can cause anaphylaxis, a severe, life-threatening condition (see pages 127–128).

### YEAST

Yeast can cause hives in adults. Avoiding yeast clears up the condition, and challenging with brewer's yeast or *Candida albicans* causes a recurrence. Chronic hives in patients who do not react directly to yeast clear up when they are put on antiyeast diets and nystatin (an antifungal medication). This suggests that their hives may be due to a sensitivity to natural yeasts (including *Candida*), that are present in the gut.

## YOGURT VERSUS YEAST

A natural treatment for yeast problems is to eat yogurt with live cultures; these usually contain a number of bacteria species, including *Lactobacillus*, which are important friendly gut bacteria. The bacteria from the yogurt may be able to outcompete and displace unfriendly gut flora, such as yeast. You can find out if the yogurt you have bought contains live cultures by following this simple procedure. Boil one cup of milk and allow it to cool. Add ½ teaspoon of the yogurt and keep the mixture in a sealed thermos for about seven hours. If the original yogurt was live, its bacteria will have converted the milk into more yogurt.

*ALIVE AND KICKING*
*If you cannot tolerate yogurt, commercial preparations of live, beneficial bacteria are available.*

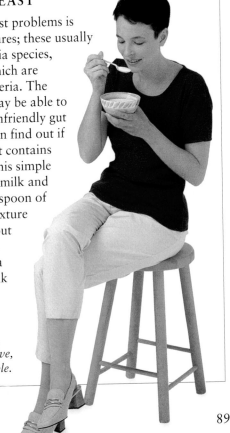

# Hypoallergenic Cooking with

# Healthy Recipes

*Egg, yeast, and wheat are commonly added to processed foods and are staple ingredients in many dishes. Fortunately, there are ways to avoid using them and still have a variety of tasty, healthy meals.*

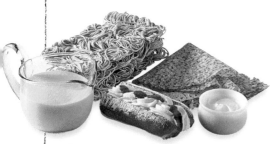

### OMNIPRESENT EGGS
*Eggs are found in cakes, cookies, muffins, pancakes, waffles, foods coated with batter, mayonnaise, and some salad dressings, ice creams, and pastas; it can be difficult to avoid them.*

Many people react with horror on being told they will have to cut out ubiquitous ingredients like egg, yeast, and wheat from their diets. However, many common dishes, such as pasta, mayonnaise, and bread, can be made without them.

### Egg-free eating
Eggs are sought after not just for their taste but also for their cooking properties. Commercial egg substitutes are available but often contain different allergens. The recipes given below for egg-free

---

### EGG-FREE MAYONNAISE

300 g (10½ oz) silken tofu
1 tbsp prepared mustard
120 ml (½ cup) olive oil
30 ml (2 tbsp) sunflower oil
1 tbsp white wine vinegar
salt and freshly ground black pepper

■ Blend the tofu and mustard in a food processor until smooth.
■ Mix the olive and sunflower oils. While the food processor is running, slowly add half the blend to the tofu mixture in a steady stream. When the mixture begins to thicken and turn pale, add the vinegar and seasoning to taste. Process until smooth.
■ Slowly blend in the remaining oil.
*Makes about 425 ml (1¾ cups)*

---

### EGG-FREE SPICY BEEF BURGERS

450 g (1 lb) lean ground beef
3 green onions
1 tbsp chopped parsley
½ tsp ground cumin
½ tsp each salt and ground black pepper

■ Chop the green onions coarsely so that there will be recognizable pieces in the cooked burgers to provide an interesting texture.
■ Place all the ingredients in a large bowl and mix until well combined.
■ Shape into four flat, round patties and grill, broil, or fry in a nonstick pan for 8 to 10 minutes, turning carefully once during cooking.
■ Serve the burgers in whole-grain pittas filled with mixed salad leaves.
*Serves 4*

---

### EGG- AND WHEAT-FREE PASTA WITH SOUR CREAM SAUCE

1 medium potato, peeled and diced
2 cloves garlic
125 g (4½ oz) low-fat sour cream
1 tbsp chopped basil
salt and freshly ground black pepper
450 g (1 lb) Jerusalem artichoke pasta

■ Bring 500 ml (2 cups) water to a boil; add the potato and garlic and simmer for 12 minutes or until the potato is tender.
■ Blend the potato, garlic, and half the cooking liquid in a food processor or blender until smooth. Add the sour cream and blend another 30 seconds.
■ Return the mixture to the pan. Stir in the basil and salt and pepper to taste. Cook over moderate heat until bubbling and thick. Pour it over the cooked pasta.
*Serves 4*

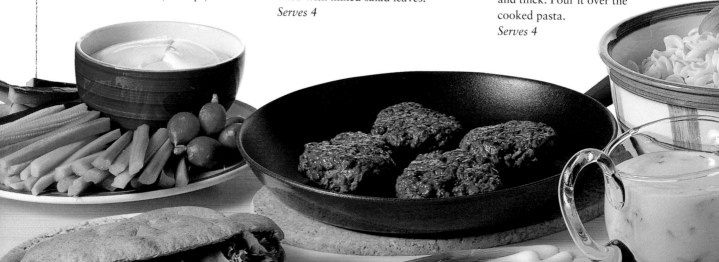

dishes show that it is possible to create a variety of delicious dishes, including some, such as mayonnaise, for which egg is usually an essential ingredient. With simple dishes like beef burgers, it is relatively easy to avoid common triggers, as long as you make them yourself. However, most people rely on processed versions, which often contain egg and egg derivatives.

## Yeast-free eating

If you have a sensitivity to yeast, you must eat yeast-free bread like Russian rye or pumpernickel or make your own loaves. The soda bread below has baking soda as the rising agent, and the cornbread is leavened with baking powder and eggs. Some flat breads, such as matzoh and tortillas, are unleavened, but others, like pitta, may have yeast added. You should also avoid wine, beer, and other alcoholic beverages, or at least moderate your intake, and other fermented products (see below right). The surface of fruit, especially dried fruit, often contains small amounts of mold, as do many nuts; if are sensitive to yeast, you should avoid these as well.

## Wheat-free eating

Thickeners and fillers are often derived from wheat, which means that a surprising number of foods can cause problems for wheat-sensitive individuals. They need to avoid most breads and many processed foods. Pastas are typically made with wheat, so a wheat-free pasta dish is included here to illustrate an alternative option.

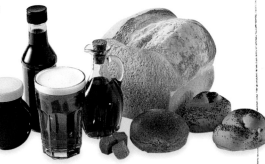

*UBIQUITOUS YEAST*
*Any food or beverage that undergoes fermentation does so because of the presence and activity of yeasts. This includes bread, soy sauce, malt, wine, vinegar, and many prepared soup stocks.*

---

### EGG-FREE STRAWBERRY ICE CREAM

2 cups crushed strawberries
225 g (1 cup) sugar
2 tsp unflavored gelatin
2 tablespoons lemon juice
480 ml (2 cups) whipping cream

- In a large bowl combine the strawberries and sugar.
- Soak the gelatin in 2 tbsp cold water until softened, then dissolve in ¼ cup boiling water. Chill until slightly thickened, then stir in the lemon juice. Stir the gelatin mixture into the fruit.
- Whip the cream until it stands in soft peaks; fold it into the fruit mixture.
- Pour into a 1-quart mold and freeze for 4 to 6 hours or until firm. Remove the ice cream from the freezer ½ hour before serving to allow it to soften.
*Makes about 1 liter (1 quart)*

---

### YEAST-FREE SODA BREAD

450 g (3½ cups) all-purpose flour
2 tsp sugar
1 tsp baking soda
1 tsp salt
1 tsp cream of tartar
300 ml (1¼ cups) milk

- Preheat the oven to 190°C/375°F.
- Sift the flour and other dry ingredients into a large bowl.
- Add the milk and mix to a soft dough, adding extra milk if needed.
- Smooth the dough by gently kneading it and shape it into a circle 3.5 cm (1½ inches) thick.
- Put the dough on a greased baking tray and score a large cross on the top
- Bake for 40 minutes.
*Makes 1 loaf*

---

### YEAST-, WHEAT-, AND MILK-FREE CORN BREAD

175 g/1 cup corn meal
25 g/3 tbsp soy flour
25 g/3 tbsp oatmeal
1 tbsp baking powder
½ tsp salt
2 eggs, beaten
240–300 ml (1–1¼ cups) soy milk
1 tbsp melted butter or margarine

- Preheat the oven to 190°C/375°F.
- Grease a 20 cm × 20 cm (8 in × 8 in) square cake pan.
- Mix the dry ingredients together. Add the eggs, soy milk, and butter or margarine and mix until smooth.
- Pour the mixture into the prepared pan and bake for about 30 minutes.
*Makes 1 loaf*

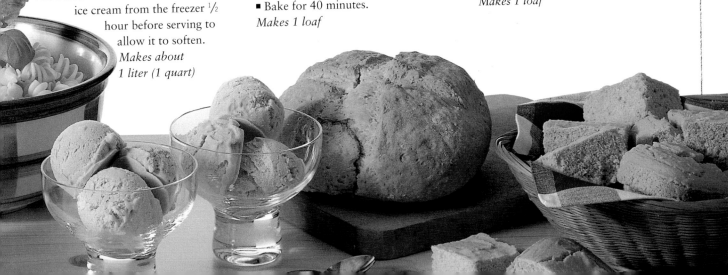

# FOODS THAT CONTAIN WHEAT, MILK, AND EGG—AND SUBSTITUTES

Avoiding the most common food allergens can be a tall order because they feature so heavily in the Western diet. They are particularly common in processed foods, where they are often difficult to spot. The chart below shows you what to look out for and suggests alternatives that might be suitable.

| TYPE OF FOOD | FOODS THAT CONTAIN WHEAT, RYE, AND BARLEY | FOODS THAT CONTAIN MILK | FOODS THAT CONTAIN EGG | SUBSTITUTES |
|---|---|---|---|---|
| Baked goods | Bread, rolls, scones, cookies, cakes, malt, cake and pastry mixes, pancakes, waffles, muffins | Some cookies, cakes, breads, and cake and pastry mixes | Some breads and rolls (especially glazed), most cakes and cookies and mixes for them, croissants | Breads and bread mixes that are milk and egg free and contain soy, lentil, buckwheat, or rice flour; plain rice cakes |
| Pasta, soups, gravies | Pastas, soups made with pasta, gravies thickened with flour | Some pasta sauces, creamed soups | Some pastas, egg noodles, noodles in some soups | Rice noodles, pure buckwheat pasta, clear soups without noodles |
| Cereals | Many breakfast cereals contain any of these or all three; some oatmeals contain added wheat. | | | Cornflakes, rice cereal, wheat-free porridge oats, wheat-free muesli, (top cereals with fruit juice or milk substitute) |
| Desserts and candy | Some pudding mixes, pies, pastries, cakes, cookies, doughnuts, ice cream cones fruit crumbles, some candies | Custard, custard powder, white sauce, pies and pastries, puddings, ice cream, milk chocolate, hot chocolate mixes | Pancakes, waffles, batters, pudding mixes, egg custard, soufflés, meringue, doughnuts, marshmallows, cakes, some ice creams | Fruit, special recipe cakes, cookies, and pastries, wheat-free batters made with alternative flours |
| Vegetables and salads | Sauces and breadcrumbs, served with vegetables or salads, croutons | Vegetables prepared with sauces or butter, some gravies and salad dressings | Scrambled and hard-cooked egg added to salads, salad dressings | All fresh, frozen, and canned vegetables, all salad ingredients |
| Meat and meat products, fish and fish products | Sausages, salami, flour used in thickening gravies and sauces for meat, breadcrumb or batter coatings, hamburgers, pies, sausage pizza, stuffing, fish fingers, fish cakes, fish in sauce or batter | Dishes cooked in butter, white sauce, milk or cheese, sausages, mortadella, Spam, gravies | Crumbed foods (for example, deep-fried fish), meat loaf and meatballs, tartar sauce, béarnaise and hollandaise sauces | All fresh fish, meat, most precooked meats if free from binders or stuffing, batters made from alternative flours, alternatives to breadcrumbs (e.g. crushed cornflakes) |
| Beverages | Drinks containing malt or barley, root beer, whisky, beer, ale | Chocolate drinks, malt drinks, some tea and coffee whiteners | Ovaltine, some instant coffees, wines that are cleared with egg white | Tea, coffee, cocoa, fruit juices, soft drinks, mineral water |
| Milk products | Commercial milk drinks, custard and custard powder, white sauce, cheese sauce, ice cream with cookie pieces | Milk, cheese, butter, most margarine, ice cream, milk powder, yogurt, buttermilk, condensed or evaporated milk | Some ice creams | Milk substitutes, tofu, vegetable purée (substitute for milk or egg), milk- and whey-free margarine |
| Ingredients of packaged and canned foods | Wheat starch, wheat flour, gluten, wheat gluten, starch, food starch, wheat germ, bran | Milk solids, skim milk, whey, milk proteins, nonfat milk, casein, caseinate, lactose | Vitellin, ovovitellin, livetin, ovomucin, ovomucoid, albumin | Check that packaged foods are free from items listed. |
| Miscellaneous | Malt vinegar, some soy sauce, communion wafers, pepper powder | | | Wine or cider vinegar, wheat-free soy sauce |

# FOOD ADDITIVES AND CONTAMINANTS

*Additives and contaminants in foods have the potential to cause allergic reactions, but they can be avoided as more organic and additive-free options become available.*

The additives and contaminants in food today come from many sources. Agricultural and industrial pollution, as well as food processing and manufacturing, all increase the unnatural substances in the things we eat and drink, whether they are added intentionally or not. Although in most cases the amounts of these substances are too small to pose any danger, continued exposure to certain chemicals may cause sensitivities in some individuals.

## CONTAMINANTS AND POLLUTION

Agriculture is the main source of contaminants in our food chain. Modern farming methods rely heavily on fertilizers and pesticides. Vast quantities of nitrates, phosphates, and other chemicals added to soil and sprayed on produce accumulate and inevitably pollute the water that runs off the land. High levels of pollutants in tap water have become a serious problem throughout the developed world.

### Pesticides and other contaminants

North American farmers use hundreds of different pesticides, which fall into three classifications: insecticides, fungicides, and herbicides. Nearly all of these can be dangerous to humans in their active state, but in theory they are sprayed onto crops long enough before harvesting to degrade before they reach the supermarket shelves. In practice, low levels of pesticides are detected in many sampled foods. And in agricultural areas, inhaled pesticides sprayed from airplanes are a major concern.

Other agricultural pollutants include the antibiotics and hormones fed to farm animals and farmed fish to make them grow faster, larger, and disease free. How many of these persist in the meat and fish that reach the dining table is not known, nor is the effect they might have. Other sources of pollution—heavy metals from industry, for instance—affect tap water. In one city in the United States low concentrations of more than 2,000 chemicals were detected in the public water supply. Domestic sources of contamination include detergents and other household chemicals, which may be carcinogenic (cancer causing).

### Are you in danger?

The food you eat probably contains only the merest traces of contaminants, but it is not possible to be sure. What's more, it is not

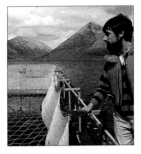

**FARMED FISH**
*Fish farms supply an increasing proportion of the fish in our diet. At some farms fish are fed heavy doses of antibiotics to fight disease.*

## AVOIDING CONTAMINANTS

The safest option is to try to avoid contaminants altogether by buying organic produce and packaged products made with organically grown foods—these are much more widely available than they were a few years ago—and drink bottled or filtered water. In addition, thorough washing or peeling can reduce the level of pollutants. (Special cleaners to remove pesticides are available in some supermarkets and health food stores.)

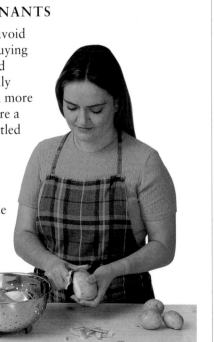

**PEEL THEM**
*Many contaminants are concentrated in or restricted to the skins of fruits and vegetables.*

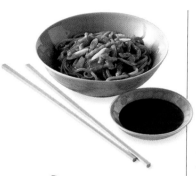

***CHINESE RESTAURANT SYNDROME***
*Monosodium glutamate (MSG) and its relatives are widely used as flavor enhancers. Large amounts of MSG are said to produce a characteristic allergic or intolerant syndrome, although the description of the symptoms varies. The use of MSG is particularly associated with food prepared in Chinese restaurants, hence the name of the syndrome. The symptoms include flushing, tightness and pain in the chest, headache, and even fainting. Although MSG has been reported to trigger attacks in some asthmatics as well, the latest evidence suggests it might not in fact be responsible for Chinese restaurant syndrome. Other ingredients, such as fermented soy sauce, are now suspected.*

really known how bad for you such traces might be. New chemicals are tested exhaustively, but there are some old ones, still in use here or in less developed countries, that were never properly tested or are, in fact, known toxins or carcinogens.

The extent to which contaminants cause allergic reactions is also unclear but some cases are known. Antibiotics in meat have caused allergic reactions, and high levels of nickel and other pollutants in tap water have caused eczema and hives.

## ADDITIVES

Few foods reach today's supermarkets free of additives—substances that do not occur naturally in food—and perhaps only a tiny minority pose any risk to health. But because additives can be found in practically anything we consume, including many medicines (in one survey 930 out of 2,204 drug formulations contained at least one additive), people who have allergies or intolerances should be aware of the variety of guises in which they might meet a trigger additive. While it is possible for any food additive to cause a problem in a sensitive individual, it appears that some cause more difficulties than others.

## Preservatives

Preservatives added to many commercially produced foods to slow their deterioration are important in the prevention of food poisoning caused by bacteria and fungi. They are essential to the modern way of processing, packaging, and transporting groceries. Fresh foods without preservatives have to be eaten within a limited period to avoid the risk of microbial contamination.

The oldest preservatives are sugar, salt, and vinegar. Manufacturers today also use many other chemicals, which fall into two groups, antimicrobials—including the benzoates, nitrates, nitrates, and sulfites—and antioxidants—ascorbic acid (vitamin C), BHA, BHT, and tocopherols (vitamin E).

## Antimicrobial preservatives

Antimicrobial preservatives extend the shelf life of foods and protect them from fungi and bacteria that can cause serious illness.

Sodium nitrate and sodium nitrite, also referred to commonly as nitrates and nitrites, are two of the most well-known and controversial preservatives; they com-

bine in the body with amines to form nitrosamines, which are toxic and carcinogenic. They are used to preserve processed meats, such as ham, bacon, sausages, hot dogs, and lunch meats, and are also added to smoked fish. Unfortunately, nitrates and nitrites can trigger symptoms such as hives and headache in susceptible individuals.

Benzoic acid and benzoates are preservatives used in fruit syrups, carbonated fruit drinks, beer, margarine, and some medicines. Benzoates also occur naturally in certain foods, particularly honey and cranberries. They have been shown to trigger hives, possibly asthma and eczema, behavioral disturbances in some hyperactive children (see page 136), and other symptoms.

Sulfites occur naturally in the fermentation of yeast. Some are always present, therefore, in wines and beers (and wine vinegars), and extra ones may be added. They are often used in the preparation of seafood, pickles, dried fruits, and dehydrated vegetables.

Sulfite sensitivity can be very difficult to detect or even to suspect. Nonetheless, asthmatics who are susceptible may react to sulfite in a food. Very sensitive asthmatics may even react to sulfur dioxide fumes from fruit juice or wines to which sulfite has been added. Sulfite sensitivity has also been shown to be a cause of other symptoms, such as rhinitis and hives.

## Antioxidant preservatives

Antioxidants prevent degradation of fats and fat-soluble vitamins. Without them fats go rancid. Butylated hydroxyanisole (BHA) and butylated hydroxytoluene (BHT) are two common antioxidants that are widely found in commercially prepared packaged foods—including potato chips, cookies, cakes, and breakfast cereals—that contain fats and oils. They can trigger hives and other symptoms in susceptible subjects.

***DRIED FRUITS***
*Some dried fruits have high levels of sulfite preservatives.*

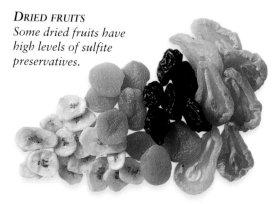

# Natural Pest Control

*Pests can easily blight your efforts to grow your own produce, but you don't have to rely on synthetic, and often toxic, chemical pesticides. Try some natural pest control methods that will keep away bugs without contaminating your food.*

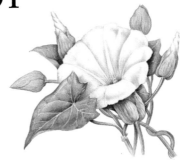

There are several ways to control pests naturally. One is to encourage friendly insects, such as ladybugs, lacewings, centipedes, and spiders, in your garden because they eat pests, like aphids and whiteflies. Another is to make insect repellents with natural ingredients.

One nontoxic remedy, widely available today for fighting pests is pyrethrin (*Pyrethrum*), derived from chrysanthemums. It kills leafhoppers, aphids, and whiteflies. An infusion of elder leaves (see below) also controls aphids. Walnut leaves boiled in water can be used as an

ant repellent. An excellent all-around insect repellent and fungicide is garlic. (To prepare it for application, purée five or six cloves with some hot chilies and two cups of water; add a few drops of liquid soap or dishwashing liquid.)

The best way to apply any of these remedies is with a spray bottle, and applications must be repeated after every rain or watering.

A lasting method for repelling aphids is to grow marigolds among your other plants, especially broad beans; marigolds attract insects like hoverflies, which prey on aphids.

**WEEDING OUT PESTS**
*Avoiding chemical weedkillers can give irritating and invasive bindweeds, such as morning glory, a chance to get a stranglehold on trees and other plants. Such plants spread quickly. Uproot and get rid of any you find in your garden.*

## COMPANION PLANTING

Companion planting involves using the proximity of a plant that is offensive to certain insects to protect other plants from their unwelcome attention. These protective plants and herbs are often strong smelling and colorful. Follow a few of the companion planting suggestions below and watch your vegetable garden flourish free from pests.

▶ *Nasturtiums should be planted with your brassicas, broad beans, and tomatoes to protect them from whiteflies and blackflies.*

▶ *French marigolds will protect tomatoes and broad beans from whiteflies and greenflies.*

▶ *Basil will repel all flying insects from your tomatoes.*

▶ *Chamomile planted among your onions will improve the yield of the crop. Onions grow faster when chamomile is present.*

▶ *A little mint planted in your cabbage patch will help fend off cabbage grubs.*

▶ *Rosemary repels carrot flies.*

## ELDER LEAF SPRAY FOR APHIDS

**1** *In a large saucepan bring 1½ liters (6 cups) of water to a boil. Add 200 g (7 oz) of fresh elder leaves (S. canadensis) and leave to steep for 10 minutes. Strain the infusion and allow it to cool.*

**2** *Fill a clean spray bottle with the infusion. Cover the entire plant with the elder spray, making sure the undersides of the leaves and stalks are thoroughly treated.*

Use a spray bottle to administer your infusions.

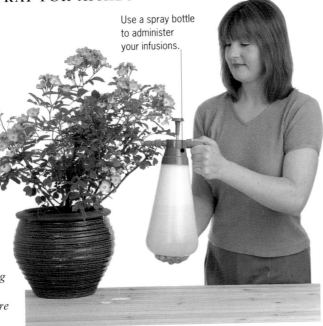

**3** *Repeat every day until the aphid infestation is cleared up. For best results, a fresh infusion should be made for each treatment. Regular treatment will keep pests away.*

## READING A FOOD LABEL

It can be difficult to identify some ingredients on a food label. Below is just a partial listing of ingredients that you might find on a packet of instant noodles, along with their sources, which could be hidden allergens.

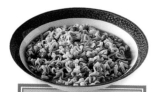

### INSTANT NOODLES
**INGREDIENTS**

Enriched wheat flour, partially hydrogenated vegetable oil, salt, hydrolyzed vegetable protein, dehydrated vegetables, monosodium glutamate, maltodextrin, caramel, yeast extract, xanthan gum, lecithin, albumen, BHA.

▶ *Hydrolyzed vegetable protein is derived from corn, soy, or wheat and sometimes all three.*

▶ *Monosodium glutamate (MSG) can provoke reactions in sensitive people; all it takes is a few milligrams.*

▶ *Dextrins and caramel are sweeteners often derived from corn.*

▶ *Lecithin is commonly derived from soybeans.*

▶ *Albumen is normally derived from egg.*

▶ *BHA (butylated hydroxyanisole) is a fat preservative that has been implicated as a cause of hives and asthma.*

## Emulsifiers, stabilizers, and thickeners

Foods that typically contain emulsifiers, stabilizers, and/or thickeners include sauces, soups, bread and other baked goods, ice cream, low-fat and nonfat sour cream and cream cheese, jams, jellies, and puddings. In addition, certain foodstuffs are used as thickeners and sweeteners in liquid medicines and as an inert base for medicinal and vitamin pills.

These additives improve the texture and consistency of processed foods by increasing smoothness, creaminess, and volume. They also hold in moisture and prevent the separation of oil and water mixtures. Common examples are carrageenan, cellulose, glycerol, guar gum, gum arabic, lecithin, and pectins. The gums can cause flatulence and abdominal pain; excessive pectin can result in bloating.

## Flavor enhancers

A number of flavorings and flavor enhancers added to foods can trigger allergic reactions. Perhaps the most well known of these is the enhancer monosodium glutamate, but allyl alcohols and other flavorings can also cause problems, even though they are used in minute amounts as a rule. Hydrolyzed vegetable protein is another flavor enhancer, used often in soup stocks.

## Food colors

Colorings, which make food products look more appetizing, are commonly used to enhance soft drinks, frostings, margarine, jams, and the skins of oranges and other fruits. Some people are sensitive to them.

In the United States the Food and Drug Administration (FDA) has tested all colorings that are permitted and designated them as GRAS (generally recognized as safe). Still, some people react to certain colors. One in particular, known as FD&C Yellow No. 5 in the United States and tartrazine in Canada, has caused problems.

What constitutes safety is sometimes open to new interpretation. Two artificial food dyes once considered safe in the United States, red 2 and violet 1, are now barred.

### RULES AND REGULATIONS

The use of food additives is governed by regulations that vary from country to country. The labeling of foods containing additives is also regulated. More than 2,800

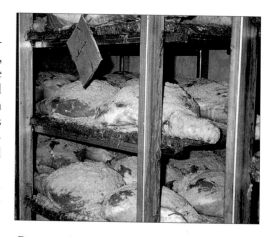

*CURE-ALL?*
*Sodium nitrate and sodium nitrite have been used in the curing of hams and bacon for centuries. In some people they can cause hives, headache, and other symptoms.*

different additives are approved for use in the United States by the FDA. Health Canada has approved 407 food additives in addition to hundreds of preservatives, colorings, flavor enhancers, and stabilizers.

## Problems with labels

Even labeling has its pitfalls, however. If a patient is sensitive to a particular preservative—BHT, for example, an antioxidant that prevents the degradation of fats—its absence on a food label might be reassuring. But what if one of the labeled ingredients—for instance, hydrogenated vegetable oil—had BHT added prior to its purchase by the food manufacturer? The presence of BHT in such circumstances might not be identified on the food label.

Another pitfall involves the words used on labels. For example, hydrolyzed vegetable protein and lecithin may both be derived from soybeans, but the word "soy" may not appear on the label. Peanut is sometimes listed as groundnut or arachis; not knowing that these terms mean "peanut" could, in extreme cases, be fatal.

## Are additives your problem?

If you have an unexplained food reaction, the best way to test the possibility that it is caused by reactions to food additives and is not a hidden allergy to the foods themselves, is to follow a diet that is totally additive free for a few weeks. You should be aware, though, that food free from overt additives may contain residues of pesticides and herbicides. You may need to use organic foods.

# EATING HEALTHFULLY WITH AN ALLERGY

*Restricting your diet to avoid triggering a food allergy need not mean that your nutrition suffers. Many people on antiallergy diets find that they are eating more healthfully than before.*

Eliminating foods from a diet because of food allergies always carries the risk of becoming deficient in some nutrients. Children on restricted diets are at particular risk, especially if they have to exclude milk, eggs, meat, or fish, which are important sources of protein; stunted growth and other signs of malnutrition may result. On the other hand, children with hidden food allergies often have a growth spurt after trigger foods are identified and avoided.

The risk of malnutrition in both children and adults results from failure to compensate for the imbalance in a restricted diet. The fewer the number of foods that can be eaten, the greater the risk that a diet will be deficient in one or more nutrients. Nonetheless, it is possible to maintain excellent nutritional intake while on a restricted diet.

## A dietitian can help

Dietitians have three useful roles in creating a balanced diet. First, they can give advice on how to avoid specific foods, by providing information on hidden sources of them. Second, they can analyze the resulting diet, often with the help of a computer, to make sure it will provide a good balance of nutrients, and they may recommend supplements, if necessary. Third, they can give suggestions on how to make the diet palatable and practical, bearing in mind that convenience is a major issue in modern life.

### MILK ALLERGY: GETTING SUFFICIENT CALCIUM

There are two compelling reasons for eliminating milk from one's diet: intolerance and allergy. Intolerance results from insufficient amounts in the body of the enzyme lactase, needed for digesting the lactose in milk, and is characterized by gas, diarrhea, cramps, and bloating after consuming milk or a milk product. More than half the adult population of the world is lactose intolerant to some degree; lactase tends to decrease with age. Milk allergy, on the other hand, is usually a reaction to the casein, lactalbumin, or lactoglobulins in milk and is manifested as a rash, eczema, wheezing, rhinitis, asthma, or anaphylaxis (in extreme cases.) A person can be both intolerant of and allergic to milk, though this is rare.

Although milk is an excellent source of calcium, it is possible to eliminate it from the diet and still obtain enough of this important mineral. Many people do not consume milk or milk products beyond early childhood and yet suffer no great degree of calcium deficiency. To be on the safe side, it is best to assume that anyone whose ancestors are from a region that normally has a high milk intake is at risk for shortage of calcium on a milk-free diet. And it should be kept in mind that the calcium needs of children, pregnant and lactating women, and women past menopause are higher than those of other people.

*MILK-FREE ZONES The orange areas on this map show the regions where the majority of adults are lactose intolerant, which includes much of the world's population.*

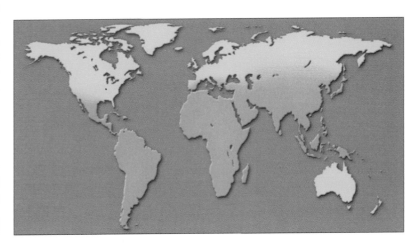

## Nondairy sources of calcium

Eliminating dairy products does not mean going without calcium. All foods provide at least a small amount of this essential mineral. The ones listed below are fairly good sources.

| FOOD | CALCIUM (mg per 100 g) | FOOD | CALCIUM (mg per 100 g) |
|---|---|---|---|
| Soft tofu | 105 | Self-rising flour | 338 |
| Roasted almonds | 300 | Cooked white beans | 73 |
| Tahini | 140 | Cooked soybeans | 146 |
| Sesame seeds, hulled | 110 | Cooked turnip greens | 137 |
| Sardines with bones | 380 | Cooked dandelions | 184 |

### Excess or deficiency?

Many patients who start an elimination diet actually improve their nutrient intake. They often reduce nonnutrients, such as refined sugar and caffeine, and eat more and a greater variety of fresh foods. Also, eliminating allergic reactions to food may improve their digestion and absorption ability, so they extract more nutrients from what they eat. It may not hurt, however, to consider taking a broadly based vitamin/mineral supplement, but it's important to seek advice first because excessive doses of some vitamins and minerals can be dangerous.

A person who has to avoid milk and milk products should compensate with other calcium-rich foods (see page 98). Calcium-enriched soy milk is a good source; many other foods are also enriched with calcium, including orange juice.

Calcium in plant foods may not be sufficient or well absorbed, and supplements may be needed as well. It's best to consult a doctor or dietitian for advice. A supplement that contains a two-to-one ratio of calcium to magnesium plus vitamin D is often recommended. In general, the calcium citrate form is more readily absorbed than other types.

Because an excess of high-protein foods, especially those rich in iron, like red meat, can speed the elimination of calcium from the system, it's best to limit their intake.

*NO MIRACLE CURES*
*Although curing your allergy can help you lose weight, you will also need to exercise and eat a sensible diet.*

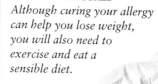

### GRAIN ALLERGY: GETTING SUFFICIENT CARBOHYDRATES

Many people have a hidden allergy to many or all of the major grains—wheat, rye, barley, oats, corn, and rice. Even if not all grains are involved (some people tolerate rice, for example, but none of the others), depending too heavily on just one grain can result in nutritional deficiencies.

For patients sensitive only to wheat, wheat-free bakery goods, breads, and other baked goods are available. These may be made with other grains, such as corn, rice, or buckwheat, or with flour made from potatoes, soybeans, or lentils. Wheat-free pasta, made with rice, buckwheat, soy, or Jerusalem artichokes is also obtainable.

People sensitive to several grains may have to use alternative sources of carbohydrates. Vegetables such as potatoes, yams, and Jerusalem artichokes are good sources of complex carbohydrates, but some vitamins or minerals may have to be supplemented.

### OBESITY AND ALLERGY

It is not unusual to find that elimination of hidden food allergens can act as an effective weight-reducing diet. Why this should happen is not clear. One possible reason is that a common symptom of hidden food allergy is fluid retention. The marked initial weight loss that occurs in people on elimination diets is almost entirely due to loss of this retained fluid. But this does not account for the sustained weight loss that often occurs.

In some patients the change of diet involves a considerable reduction in calories (if, for example, they were previously eating a lot of foods containing sugar). In others this is not the case, but it may be that improvement in health and well-being leads to an increase in the general level of exercise. This in turn burns off calories and raises an individual's metabolic rate—the rate at which they burn up calories—decreasing weight even further.

It is also possible that in some patients food allergens directly affect their weight-regulating mechanism in some way, affecting weight control adversely by a means other than calorie buildup. This is a tempting hypothesis for those who fail to lose weight with calorie restriction. However, for nonallergic people, lack of exercise and failure to follow a balanced diet are more likely to be the culprits.

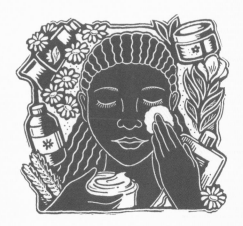

# CHAPTER 5

# CONTACT ALLERGIES AND OTHER SKIN REACTIONS

*Disorders of the skin are among the most common problems that physicians have to deal with, and conventional medicine has developed a battery of drugs to treat them. But this is one area in which alternative remedies and therapies can be really helpful. Natural strategies for controlling and managing skin problems can help reduce the need for drugs or even make them unnecessary.*

# SKIN REACTIONS AND THEIR CAUSES

*The skin can reflect many conditions in the body, from illness to food allergy to contact dermatitis. Finding the exact cause of a skin eruption is often challenging.*

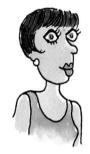

*THICK SKINNED?*
*People's sensitivity to irritants varies with age; it is greatest in children, lessens in early adult life, but then increases again with old age. Skin type makes a difference too.*

**Brunettes** have less vulnerable skin than blondes.

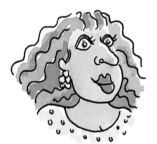

**Redheads** have the most vulnerable skin.

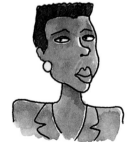

**Black skin** is probably the most resistant to irritants.

Rashes can be symptomatic of many problems, including illnesses like measles, chickenpox, or streptococcal sore throat; reactions to foods or inhaled allergens; and reactions to contact with a toxin—stinging nettles, poison ivy, or irritant chemicals, for instance. Particularly sensitive individuals may react also to a drug—penicillin is a common trigger—and can develop contact reactions from substances that are harmless to others. These include some plants and animals, house dust mites, nickel in jewelry, the fiber content or finishes of some fabrics and carpets, and exposure to certain chemicals.

Anyone may develop skin problems occasionally, but some people have more sensitive skin than others and are constantly plagued. People who continually have skin reactions are considered hyperreactive, and they may even develop rashes as a result of emotional stress or exposure to sunlight or cold. If a sufferer can avoid particular allergens much of the time, this hypersensitivity may gradually lessen.

## DIFFERENT TYPES OF SKIN REACTIONS

The range of terms used to describe skin problems can be confusing. The main terms are hives, eczema, and dermatitis.

Hives (also called nettle rash and urticaria) is a very itchy condition that exhibits reddening of the skin and whitish bumps, most often small but sometimes as much as an inch or more across. The condition is usually short lasting but may appear in a series of waves, going on for months. Hives affect the middle layers of the skin, but may also involve the deeper layers, resulting in swelling that is called angioedema.

Eczema is a chronic type of skin rash that develops more slowly and is generally less itchy than hives. "Atopic eczema" is the term used for the condition in patients who have atopy—the general predisposition for developing such allergic reactions as hives, asthma, rhinitis, and Type A food allergy. However, the term "eczema" is also used for rashes that are not caused by an allergy.

Housewife's hand eczema refers to the dry, rough, and reddened skin on the hands of anyone who constantly uses detergents, household cleaners, and shampoos. People whose hands are exposed to chemicals in the workplace may also develop this condition

Dermatitis is a broader term that covers conditions due either to irritation or allergens, and it is also used for some other skin problems. Contact dermatitis describes any skin reaction provoked by contact with an irritant or allergen.

### ALLERGY VERSUS IRRITATION

An irritant is a substance, like a solvent in paint or a toxin in a plant, that breaks through the protective outer layers of the skin and causes damage and irritation. The irritation can, in turn, make the skin more vulnerable to infection or, in allergic individuals, sensitize the skin so that the irritant or another substance will in the future produce an allergic reaction.

Although some people are more sensitive to irritants than others, some chemicals or toxins are usually harmful to anyone's skin. In contrast, certain "contact allergens," like latex, may be completely harmless to the majority of individuals. Even in allergic people, their effects are likely to be delayed, from a few hours to two days—making it hard to identify what is acting as a trigger.

## WHO IS SUSCEPTIBLE?

Eczema in an infant is one of the first signs of atopy, a generalized tendency to hypersensitivity, which is at least partly genetic in origin. This means that a tendency to develop skin allergy may be inherited and that children of allergic parents are more at risk. As with other allergic conditions, environmental factors in the early years of life also play an important role.

Even infants or young children who are not prone to allergies may develop skin problems temporarily because their skin is very tender. Contact allergies are also more common in older people because their skin tends to thin and weaken with age.

### The state of your skin

Dry, broken, cut, or abraded skin is more susceptible to allergens and irritants. Disorders that produce some of these conditions, therefore, increase susceptibility to skin allergies. For instance, people with ichthyosis, in which the skin is abnormally dry, are very vulnerable, and their skin condition requires constant moisturizing. Such people can also benefit from taking a vacation in the humidity of the tropics. On the other hand, they have to be careful about sweat; it can make the skin more vulnerable because it spreads some allergens—nickel from buttons for instance.

Other influences on the skin include smoking and excessive exposure to sunlight and harsh weather, especially extremes of

## HOW IRRITATION AND ALLERGY DIFFER

The distinctions between allergy and irritation reflect the different ways in which they cause damage to the skin; allergy occurs only when there is an immune system response.

| | IRRITATION | ALLERGY |
|---|---|---|
| Cause of symptoms/ condition | Direct damage from irritant | Reaction to low concentrations of a normally harmless substance |
| Who is vulnerable? | Everyone, although people's skins vary in toughness | Minority of people who have been sensitized |
| Long-term effects | Skin may harden and become resistant, but most damage heals without lasting scars | Skin remains sensitive to very low concentrations of an allergen. Allergic skin reactions may be chronic—lasting for a long time—or they may be recurrent. |

temperature. Any of these can dry out the skin, alter its pH balance, and generally make it more vulnerable.

### Nutrition and skin

Nutrition is a crucial factor in skin health. The lipid content of the top layer of the skin has to be maintained at a healthy level. Deficiencies in diet or a poorly functioning metabolism can compromise this, but a diet rich in essential fatty acids (EFA) and the antioxidant vitamins A, C, and E can help to guard against skin problems. There is evidence also that evening primrose oil, which is rich in the EFA gamma-linolenic acid, can help heal eczema (see page 108).

## THE SKIN'S DEFENSES

Skin is composed of two main layers—the epidermis, which provides the body's first line of defense against hostile organisms and substances, and the dermis. Lying beneath these two is a layer of subcutaneous fat.

**The epidermis** has a top layer of dead cells filled with a protein called keratin, set in a matrix of lipids (fats and oils). The keratin layer is the main defense against irritants, and it can also withstand a lot of mechanical and chemical damage.

**The dermis** is composed mainly of dense but springy collagen, a protein that gives skin its elasticity and shock-absorbing capacity. Running through the dermis are many blood vessels, which help with temperature regulation.

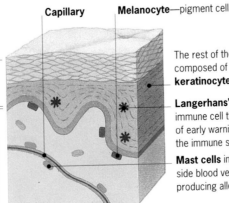

**Capillary**

**Melanocyte**—pigment cell

The rest of the epidermis is composed of live cells called **keratinocytes**.

**Langerhans' cell** is a type of immune cell that acts as a sort of early warning for the rest of the immune system.

**Mast cells** in the dermis and alongside blood vessels are involved in producing allergic skin responses.

# COMMON SYMPTOMS OF SKIN ALLERGIES

*Itching, redness, and swelling are common features of allergic skin reactions. Understanding the course of a condition is a vital first step toward coping with and treating such symptoms.*

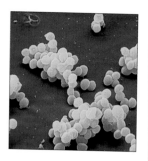

**STAPHYLOCOCCUS AUREUS**
*The staphylococcus bacterium, seen here under a scanning electron microscope, is a common invader of broken skin, such as that produced by scratching. It can worsen inflammation and irritation.*

**SYMPTOMS AND LAYERS**
*Different symptoms and effects are produced in the skin, according to which layer is affected.*

Disorders of the top layer produce eczema or dermatitis.

Disorders of the middle layer produce hives (urticaria).

If problems spread to the subcutaneous layer, severe swelling (angioedema) results.

Skin reactions exhibit a set of common symptoms, as well as symptoms that are particular to each condition. Characteristic reactions include redness (erythema), accompanied by raised bumps (wheals) and blisters (vesicles) of fluid, which may ooze or join together to form larger blisters. The skin itches at various intensities, and scratching gives rise to a further set of consequences.

## ECZEMA AND DERMATITIS

Eczema and some forms of dermatitis are chronic conditions involving redness and inflammation of the skin, which tends to thicken and become rough and flaky. Severity varies; increased itchiness is often a sign that the condition is getting worse. The severity of itching ranges from minimal to moderate, and occasionally is severe. If the condition is acute, tiny bubbles or vesicles develop; these may coalesce to form blisters, which may then burst and weep.

Chronic forms involve dryness of the skin and flaking on the surface, which becomes steadily thicker until deep fissures form. These are painful and may bleed. Intermediate forms between the two extremes are common. Dermatitis heals without scarring or residual damage, even after a chronic episode lasting for years.

More than one mechanism and any part of the body may be involved, and the area covered may be small or extensive. The hands are affected in 50 percent of cases. If the whole body surface is involved, a condition known as erythroderma, the consequences can be serious, including a breakdown in the mechanism that regulates body temperature. The result may be excessive loss of heat, dehydration, mineral depletion, and in the elderly, heart failure.

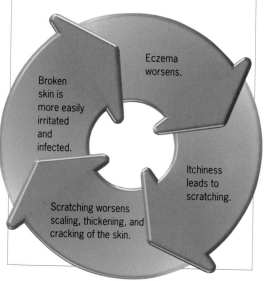

### THE VICIOUS CYCLE OF SCRATCHING

Once skin is broken, it becomes more vulnerable to irritants, allergens, and infection by invasive bacteria.

Eczema worsens.

Itchiness leads to scratching.

Scratching worsens scaling, thickening, and cracking of the skin.

Broken skin is more easily irritated and infected.

## Childhood eczema

Mostly affecting children of allergic parents, eczema usually starts in the first year of life, sometimes within a few days of birth, and it often doesn't clear up until puberty. It may affect the face, body, limbs, or crotch area and localize in the flexures (insides of the elbows and back of the knees) during the second year. Flexural eczema is often caused by foods, most often milk and eggs, but children with eczema should not be put on elimination diets without medical supervision and precautions; serious reactions may occur after challenges. Eczema on the outer side of the limbs is more likely to result from contact with dust mite allergens or chemicals found on carpets. Small children must be allowed to crawl, however, so protect them with long cotton rompers and long-sleeved tops and wash their garments often.

## Eczema in adults

In adults, eczema is usually divided into two types: exogenous eczema, meaning it is caused by something outside the body—by allergy or irritation—and idiopathic, which means it is of unknown origin. Some forms of eczema are regarded as nonallergies because no cause has been identified. In such a case, a number of triggers may be involved, so avoiding only one of them usually makes little difference. Other types, such as hypostatic eczema in the elderly, are definitely not allergies

### ACNE COSMETICA

Sometimes adults suddenly develop spots and blemishes on their faces, usually around 20 or 30 years of age. These are caused by cosmetics, soaps, or shaving creams. The condition more commonly affects women. Many cosmetics and cleansing products contain ingredients that can irritate the skin and cause allergic reactions. The simplest treatment is to stop using any product that causes a problem, but sufferers may have sensitive skin that also needs special care.

### HIVES

Also known as urticaria and nettle rash, hives are often, but not always, caused by an allergic reaction. They can result from direct skin contact with either a toxin, such as poison oak, ivy, or sumac, or an allergen, or by ingesting or inhaling an allergen. For instance, hives are a classic consequence of an allergic reaction to nuts or shellfish.

An itchy red rash appears on the skin and localized swellings develop, caused by blood vessels leaking plasma (the watery part of the blood) into the surrounding tissue. These appear as raised white spots on a red background and are known as wheals.

## Angioedema

About 50 percent of people with hives develop angioedema, also known as angioneurotic edema. This condition is characterized by swelling of deeper tissues. It affects particularly the lips, eyes, and genital area. Angioedema can

be serious if it affects the tongue or throat, and medical help should be sought speedily because suffocation may result.

## Acute and chronic hives

An acute case of hives causes intense itching that comes on quickly and usually goes away within 24 hours, though it can last for a few days. The condition can be caused by foods, a hyperreaction to insect bites or stings, drugs like penicillin, or substances that come in contact with the skin. It may be accompanied by nausea and fever, in which case the term "anaphylaxis" is more appropriate (see page 127). Because symptoms appear so rapidly, the condition can often be linked to an obvious cause, which should be avoided in the future.

Chronic hives are much more difficult to pin down, and some sufferers never learn what triggers their condition. Hives can last for months or even years—not continually, but constantly appearing and then fading on different parts of the body. In some patients the problem is linked with food triggers, though not necessarily food allergy. Some foods, like fish and sauerkraut, are naturally high in histamine, and in individuals who do not readily break down histamine this may trigger symptoms directly, but it is not the same as an allergy. In other patients hives seem to result from abnormal populations of organisms in the gut, such as fungi. For these people a diet low in fermented foods and sugars and that includes yogurt with live cultures can be helpful.

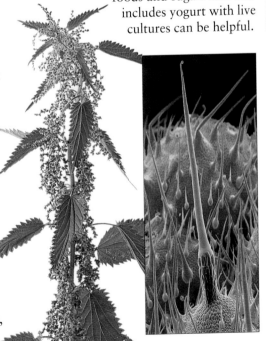

*STINGING NETTLE*
*Hives, or urticaria, is also known as nettle rash because the stinging nettle, Urtica dioica, causes the same reaction on contact with the skin. The surfaces of nettle leaves are covered with sharp, hollow hairs that contain histamine.*

# COMMON ALLERGENS AND IRRITANTS

*Anyone with sensitive skin is probably keenly aware of the potential dangers posed by cosmetics, soaps, fabrics, and other products encountered in daily life.*

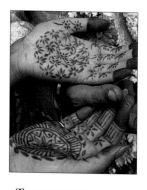

***TRADITIONAL MAKEUP***
*An Indian girl uses henna, a plant pigment, to trace designs on the palms of her hands. Pigments derived from plants and minerals have been used for millennia.*

***OVERALL COVER***
*Some of the chemicals used in gardening can provoke a skin reaction. Gardeners may also need to protect themselves from the saps of pine trees and other plants.*

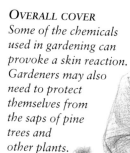

The 20th century saw a startling rise in the incidence of eczema, dermatitis, and hives. It is entirely possible that prehistoric men and women suffered from skin irritation due to toxic pigments, metal ornaments, and rough fabrics, but contact allergies are a relatively modern phenomenon. What has changed? The cosmetics and other personal products we use today include a huge number of artificial compounds. Artificial and often highly potent chemicals are also now in everyday use in a variety of domestic and occupational settings.

## PLANTS

The classical triggers of contact rashes and hives are nettles, poison oak, poison ivy, and poison sumac. (The last three are especially widespread in North America.) All these plants have defense mechanisms that cause a skin reaction in anyone who touches them, but poison oak, ivy, and sumac can produce a rash just by touching clothing or pets that have been in contact with the plants or being exposed to smoke from the plants when burned. For some people the consequences can be severe, with a widespread and long-lasting rash.

Juices in plant stems and saps in trees can act as irritants or allergens also; some interact with sunlight to cause the reaction known as phototoxic dermatitis. Many of the chemicals used in gardening can trigger reactions as well; it is important to wear gloves when handling them and wear long sleeves and pants when working in the garden.

## PERSONAL PRODUCTS

There are so many potential triggers in cosmetics and personal products like shampoo, deodorant, hair dye, mouthwash, and skin creams, it is impossible to list them all. Common culprits are dyes, preservatives, and fragrances. If a cosmetic causes a reaction, you can probably find another one with different ingredients that won't. Hypoallergenic products may be better tolerated because they are often made with ingredients that cause the fewest problems.

## FOODS

Food allergies are a common cause of both acute and chronic skin problems. The reaction may occur on contact, causing an outbreak on the lips and in the mouth, or it may appear after the food reaches the stom-

### OCCUPATIONAL EXPOSURE

Contact dermatitis is the most common occupational disorder. Millions of working days are lost annually in the United States and Canada because of this complaint. Mainly the hands are affected, and some professions are more hazardous than others. Caterers, cleaning people, hairdressers, workers in manufacturing that involves chemicals, and mechanics are all at risk because they have so much contact with hot water, detergents, and various chemicals.

ach. It is possible that more than half of childhood eczema is due to food allergy. The main food allergens are milk, eggs, wheat, soy, peanuts, tree nuts, and seafood. Such additives as colorings, flavorings, and preservatives can also cause reactions.

## WATER

Prolonged exposure to water, especially hot water, can break down the protective lipid outer barrier of the epidermis and cause chapping. This makes the skin more vulnerable to further reactions. Using cotton-lined rubber gloves helps protect the skin.

## RUBBER

The latex in rubber can cause allergies, with reactions ranging from mild eczema to full-blown anaphylaxis (see page 127). Latex is used in diaphragms, condoms, rubber bands, and disposable gloves. The last are worn in the health care industry and occupations involving the handling of hazardous substances (about 10 percent of people in such occupations are at risk). Patients who undergo many surgical procedures are particularly susceptible to latex allergy.

The powder used to lubricate gloves sometimes carries latex particles into the air, where they can trigger rhinitis. Alternative gloves made of vinyl or a synthetic are available but are more expensive.

Individuals with latex allergy may also react to foods that contain some of the same proteins found in latex. These foods include bananas, avocados, and kiwifruit.

## SOAPS AND DETERGENTS

Detergents bond with fats and oils, allowing them to be washed away. As a result, prolonged exposure to detergents will also strip the skin of its protective fats and oils. Eczema sufferers should avoid using soap altogether or use a mild, nonperfumed soap and follow bathing with emollients. (Sensitive people may also react to contaminants in tap water when washing; installing a filter with an activated carbon element in the water system or showerhead can help.)

Some laundry detergents cause problems that may be due to the formula or added enzymes or perfumes. By experimenting with different brands, most sufferers can find a washing product they can tolerate. Putting clothes through two rinses or a second wash cycle without any detergent can

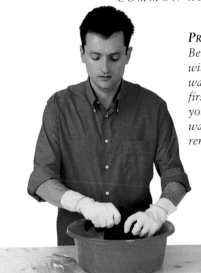

*PREWASH*
*Because new clothes are often treated with chemicals, it is a good idea to wash them before wearing them the first time. For hand washables protect your hands with rubber gloves and wash your hands immediately after removing the gloves.*

help. If none of the above approaches work, clothes can be washed with baking soda or borax. Fabric softeners should be avoided because these, too, can cause reactions.

## CLOTHING AND FABRICS

Allergy sufferers are often unable to tolerate new clothes. They may be reacting to the fiber, the finishes, or the dyes. Wool and cotton can sometimes act as allergens, but in general, artificial fibers cause the most problems, especially polyester, viscose, and rayon. Skin allergy sufferers should wear loose cotton clothing and use pure cotton bedding; linen or silk are possible alternatives.

## METALS

Nickel is a common cause of allergy, probably because of its widespread use in jewelry, watchbands, clothing fasteners, eyeglass frames, and coins. The prevalence of ear piercing among women may explain why they more often react to nickel than men do.

Two other troublesome metals are chromium and copper. Intrauterine devices made from copper can cause problems for women who use them. Anyone who is having orthodonture work done may have an allergic reaction to metal bands because they often contain chromium, copper, and/or nickel.

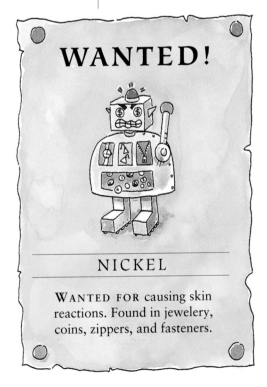

# WANTED!

## NICKEL

**WANTED FOR** causing skin reactions. Found in jewelry, coins, zippers, and fasteners.

## DRUG-FREE ITCH RELIEF

The basic principles of drug-free relief from itching are keeping the skin cool and moist and avoiding irritation. Simple measures include rubbing ice cubes on the skin and applying cold, wet compresses. You can make these out of crushed ice cubes wrapped in a washcloth. Dressings like this help cool inflammation, relieve itching, and prevent oozing and weeping. Follow up cold compresses with calamine lotion or a dressing of zinc oxide paste, available from pharmacies. A cool bath with the addition of oil, such as olive or a few drops of aromatherapy oil, oatmeal, baking powder, or cornstarch can help to soothe and rehydrate the skin. A little vinegar in water also soothes and helps restore the correct pH balance (6–7) of the skin. Avoid soap or use nonperfumed, mild soaps in the bath and moisturize your skin afterward with gentle, nonperfumed lotion or cream. Other recommendations are to use cotton clothing and sheets, stay out of the sun, and keep cool. Also, try to maintain a constant but moderate level of humidity in the house.

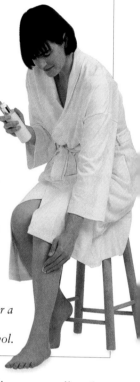

*KEEP MOIST*
*Your skin can dry out after a bath, so use a moisturizer without fragrance or alcohol.*

### NATURAL TREATMENTS

Effective natural alternatives are worth exploring. Relieving itchiness and preventing the negative cycle of scratching and damage is the first step. Some treatments may go deeper.

### Evening primrose oil (EPO)

Deficiencies in the intake and processing of essential fatty acids (EFAs) have been linked to eczema (see page 101). Evening primrose oil is rich in EFAs and has been shown to improve eczema. A 1982 study on 60 adults and 39 children at the Bristol Royal Infirmary in England showed improvement in itching after taking evening primrose oil for 12 weeks. EPO is available both over the counter and by prescription.

### Chinese medicine

The herbal remedies that have been used for centuries in traditional Chinese medicine have sparked interest because of claims that they can cure severe, chronic atopic dermatitis. Conventional Western medicine has failed to conquer this condition. The patients who seem to derive the most benefit from Chinese medicine are those who are not severely affected, but the same holds true for almost any medical treatment. Practitioners of Chinese medicine also prescribe remedies for treating hives.

Chinese herbal remedies are usually taken as decoctions—infused in boiling water like a tea. These teas can be extremely unpleasant to drink, and more palatable freeze-dried preparations of the complex mixtures are available by prescription. The remedies appear to be effective in about half of cases. However, the action of the herbs is not well understood, and there is known to be a risk of kidney or liver damage due to lack of control and regulation of potentially toxic ingredients. Any patient taking this treatment should be thoroughly monitored by a doctor, as well as an herbalist.

### Other alternative remedies

Opinions are divided over the benefits of homeopathy in eczema treatment, but there are several remedies commonly used for hives, including *Apis mellifica*, *Urtica urens* and *Dulcamara*.

Naturopathy is a good option to consider because food allergies are common triggers of both hives and dermatitis.

Herbal remedies applied to the skin can be useful; calendula, chickweed, and aloe vera ointments can help with soreness, dryness, and itching. Chamomile lotion can aid in relieving the inflammation of hives. All of these herbal options should be used with caution in case you are allergic or sensitive to the plants or their close relatives.

### Cooling foods

In Chinese medicine cooling foods are recommended to nourish the yin and disperse the hot yang energy in order to reduce irritation. A naturopath may pursue the same effect by prescribing a raw food diet that excludes all sweet foods, even honey and dried fruits.

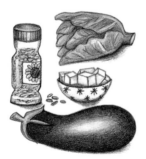

*STAY COOL*
*Cooling foods include sunflower seeds, eggplant, lettuce, and tofu.*

# PREVENTING SKIN ALLERGIES

*Prevention is always better than treatment, and treating skin allergies is often difficult. Taking care of your skin by following basic precautions can help you to stay healthier.*

Extreme conditions are the enemy of sensitive skin. Excessive heat can cause inflammation, as well as sweating, and the sweating in turn can irritate skin and block the pores. Exposure to cold, windy weather can cause chapping and cracking and strip skin of its protective properties. Prolonged contact with water, (especially hot water) astringent soaps, or rough clothing can also cause damage.

### AVOIDING EARLY EXPOSURE

When there is a family history of allergies, taking precautions during late pregnancy and the first year of an infant's life can reduce the incidence of eczema. Mothers should consider avoiding excessive amounts of allergenic foods like milk, eggs, fish, and nuts, and any foods to which they themselves are sensitive, both during the last three months of pregnancy and during lactation. They should also consider not giving their infants eggs, fish, wheat, or citrus fruits until past the age of nine months and

take steps to reduce exposure to house dust mites. It may help for a mother to take supplements of vitamins, minerals—using a product designated especially for pregnancy and lactation)—and evening primrose oil, which is rich in essential fatty acids. Young babies are more likely to develop eczema if their mother's milk is low in essential fatty acids. Be careful, too, about exposing an infant to chemicals and other allergens, such as pets and high pollen counts. In particular, you should not allow your child's sensitive skin to come in contact with harsh detergents and synthetic fabrics.

### TREATING YOUR SKIN GENTLY

The first rule of good skin care is to treat your skin gently. Basic beauty and skin-care guidelines apply here. Both men and women with sensitive skin should follow much the same rules as apply to those who are seeking to avoid wrinkles.

Avoid overexposure to the sun and protect yourself from its damaging rays with sunscreens. Remember to take care when choosing a sun lotion: sunscreens may contain substances like PABA (para-amino benzoic acid), cinnamon oil, or fragrances that can provoke a reaction.

Prevent your skin from drying out by using mild, nonfragranced, hypoallergenic soap, moisturizers, and emollients and try to reduce the number of baths and showers you take. Pat yourself dry after washing, rather than rubbing. Be particularly aware of the moisture of your skin in dry climates (hot or cold) and rooms with air conditioning.

Use simple cosmetics and body-care products to minimize the number of ingredients that come into contact with your skin. Once you have found a cosmetic or other

**BIOHAZARDS**
*Watch out for extreme conditions that can dry or chafe your skin.*

Heat increases the severity of inflammation and makes you sweat—itself an irritant.

Dryness robs your skin of protective moisture, making it vulnerable to cracking.

Immersing your skin in water for long periods of time can strip it of protective oils.

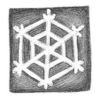

Extreme cold can cause chapping, especially in windy or wet conditions.

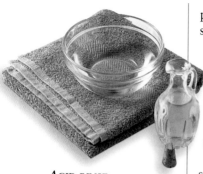

*ACID RINSE*
*Rinsing your skin with vinegar water—60 ml (2 tbsp) in 1 liter (1 quart) of water—can help maintain your skin's correct pH level.*

personal product that works well for you, stick with it, but be aware that as people grow older they can develop allergies or intolerances to products they have used for many years.

To protect your skin's pH level use mildly acidic soaps or apply special ointments, for instance, those that contain urea, or try a vinegar rinse (see recipe, left).

If you are trying a new product, use it sparingly at first and keep an eye out for any warning signs or early symptoms of a reaction. The sooner you stop exposing your skin to an irritant or allergen, the less damage will be done and the easier it will be to recover. Remember, though, that not having a reaction to it at first does not mean you will not become allergic or sensitive to that substance later on.

### STRESS AND RELAXATION

The health of your skin is regarded as a key indicator of mental health, particularly for people with sensitive skin. In fact, skin has been described as the window on the body because of the way in which it shows telltale signs of illness and changes in emotions. Stress, depression, and fatigue can cause or exacerbate skin reactions of all sorts; hives, in particular, are made worse by stress. Part of the stress response is a heightened awareness of irritations such as itchiness, so that stressed people may scratch more, thus worsening skin conditions.

A healthy mind can have a direct, positive influence on your immune system, on the levels in your blood of inflammatory substances, like histamine, and anti-inflammatory substances, like prostaglandins, and on your general ability to fight disease.

After finding and avoiding the triggers of your hives or dermatitis, the most effective step you can take toward controlling and minimizing it may be to reduce the level of stress in your life and learn to cope with stress more effectively (see page 73 for breathing techniques that release stress).

> **WARNING**
> *Never do a self-test with any strong or concentrated chemical and never apply a test substance to skin that is inflamed, sore, or cracked.*

## SELF-ADMINISTERING A PATCH TEST

If you have an unexplained skin reaction, or if you know that you have sensitive skin and are worried about the possible effect of a newly encountered product, you can try a patch test to check. You should allow 48 hours for the test.

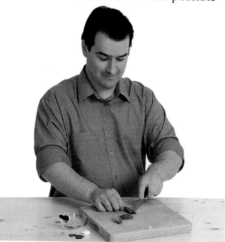

**1** *Use a sterile strip or bandage to hold a sample of the substance—a piece of cloth, a leaf fragment, or a household or personal product at the concentration it would normally be used—in place on your forearm.*

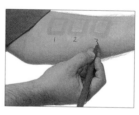

**2** *Use a pen to code each substance on your skin, after checking that the ink itself does not produce a reaction. If a test site begins to itch, take the sterile strip off and consider the test positive.*

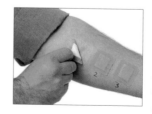

**3** *Remove the strips after 48 hours, wait for an hour because the skin may be moist, and then look and feel for raised or red skin. Check again one and two days later. If a reaction has occurred, avoid contact with that substance.*

# CHAPTER 6

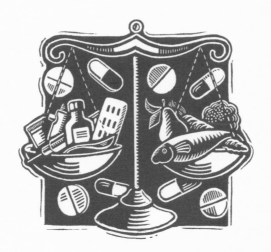

# DRUG ALLERGIES

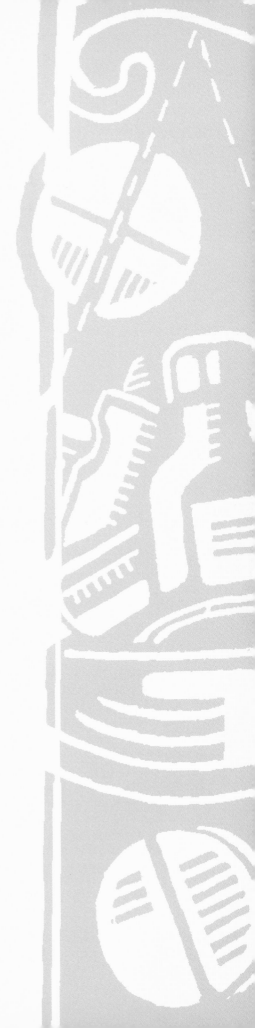

*The development of thousands of new drugs and the increasingly widespread use of antibiotics have led to a dramatic upsurge in allergic reactions to medications. There are many ways to avoid the problems of drug allergy, however, and in learning to manage your allergy, you may also make dramatic improvements to your health.*

# ALLERGIES AND OTHER SIDE EFFECTS

*Many medications have unwanted side effects, but in sensitive individuals certain drugs—including some of the most widely used ones—can produce a potentially serious allergic reaction.*

The role of a medication is, of course, to relieve symptoms and alter the course of an illness. Ideally a drug will work in a beneficial way; if it is an antibiotic, it will help fight an invader. But drugs can also have a number of adverse effects. When they result from a reaction of the immune system to the drug, it is said to be an allergic side effect.

### SIDE EFFECTS

Responses produced by a drug that are neither intended nor therapeutic are said to be side effects. There are three main types.

## Pharmacological side effects

Pharmacological side effects, produced by direct action of a drug on the body, can be pleasant or unpleasant. For instance, some antibiotics cause diarrhea. This does not help them to work and is an unwanted side effect that varies in severity from patient to patient. An example of a drug with a good side effect is minoxidil. At first (and still) prescribed to treat high blood pressure, it was discovered to stimulate hair growth in balding people, and it is now prescribed topically for that purpose.

## Toxic side effects

The difference between a therapeutic effect and a toxic one is often just a matter of degree—sometimes based on the size of the dose—and tolerances can vary from person to person. A toxic drug dose is damaging rather than therapeutic. Licensing authorities usually demand a large safety margin between a prescribed dose and the lowest dose that is likely to cause serious harm.

## Allergic side effects

Allergic side effects occur when a patient's immune system reacts to a drug and an allergic response follows. This response may result in a variety of symptoms, from a rash to wheezing to full-blown anaphylaxis.

### LEVELS OF SUSCEPTIBILITY

People differ in their susceptibility to unwanted pharmacological and toxic effects of drugs. For instance, some elderly patients cannot tolerate doses that would be safe for younger people. Anyone who is deficient in certain nutrients is also more susceptible to harmful effects caused by normally safe drug doses. At the extreme end of the spectrum, allergic individuals may suffer side effects from tiny amounts of a drug—doses far lower than those that would cause problems for someone who is not allergic.

## TOXIN TOLERANCE

Grigory Rasputin, a mysterious figure at the court of Tsar Nicholas II of Russia, is an extraordinary example of how people's tolerance for toxins can vary considerably. He was assassinated by Russian aristocrats, worried by his influence at court, and in their initital attempt survived drinking enough cyanide to kill several men. Rasputin was finally drowned in the icy River Neva. Some believe his heavy drinking habits may have contributed to his unusual resistance to cyanide.

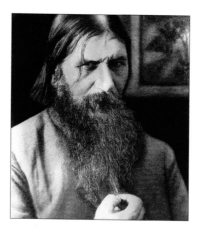

*GRIGORY RASPUTIN (1872–1916) Confidant of the last Russian Tsarina, Rasputin was incredibly resistant to the toxic effects of cyanide.*

# SYMPTOMS OF DRUG ALLERGIES

*Drug allergies are of serious concern to physicians, who must be alert to telltale signs of danger so that they can protect their patients and find effective alternative treatments.*

A number of symptoms are associated with drug allergy, but unfortunately they cannot be used as an infallible guide to whether the reaction is an allergic or nonallergic one. Doctors must use a blend of experience and careful scrutiny of a patient's history to determine whether allergies are to blame. The most severe reactions to a drug are likely to occur when a person's immune system produces the allergic antibody IgE (see page 16)

### SKIN RASHES

The most common allergic reaction to a drug is a measles-like rash, which usually appears within the first few days of treatment. Drug rashes can occur with either topical or systemic preparations.

Hives, or uticaria, is another common reaction. Sometimes the bumps are large and joined together, and the rash may be accompanied by areas of swelling, usually around the mouth, eyes, and neck, known as angioedema. But not all rashes related to medications result from allergies. In particular, those associated with bleeding into the skin, which may appear as small red dots that are not obvious to the nonspecialist, are not usually allergic in nature.

### NAUSEA AND BOWEL PROBLEMS

Some medications cause dizziness and blurred vision, which in turn may lead to nausea, but these are rarely the result of allergic reactions. Bowel disturbances and discomfort, which include cramps and constipation or diarrhea, can occur as a result of allergy, but they are more often a nonallergic side effect, caused, for example, by preparations of iron given to combat anemia or peptic ulcers; they can also indicate an inability to tolerate a particular drug.

### HEADACHES AND FATIGUE

Such vague and generalized reactions as lethargy, fatigue, and headaches, all common responses to drugs, are sometimes allergic in nature. They can be caused by minute quantities of a drug. However, these symptoms tend to be underreported, and so doctors cannot respond to them.

### PHOTOSENSITIVITY

Allergy to drugs can make skin sensitive to bright sunlight, which will cause it to become red and sore like an exaggerated sunburn. The condition sometimes persists for decades and may be extremely disabling. Sufferers have to cover up, wear sunblock (which itself may provoke an irritant or allergic reaction), and stay out of the sun. Long-term exposure to tetracyclines, used to control teenage acne, can cause this condition.

### ANAPHYLAXIS

Allergy to penicillin and antibiotics in the same family, including amoxicillin and ampicillin, is one of the leading causes of anaphylaxis, the most severe form of allergic reaction. Injections are more likely to cause anaphylaxis than drugs taken orally.

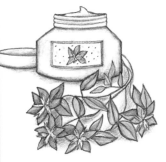

**CHICKWEED OINTMENT**
*Herbalists recommend chickweed ointment for natural relief from the itchiness of hives.*

**COVER UP**
*Photosensitive people have to cover up, wear hypoallergenic sunblock, and stay out of the sun.*

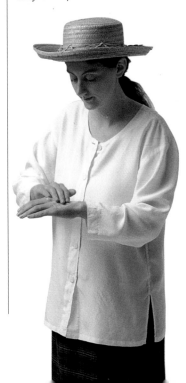

---

> ### WARNING
> *Urticaria (hives) and angioedema can be followed by more severe allergic reactions if the same drug is taken again. Angioedema can also become dangerous if your throat swells up. See your doctor immediately if you notice sudden swelling of your tongue or throat.*

# COMMON PROBLEM DRUGS

*Most drug allergies are caused by a few commonly used drugs. Antibiotics are the main culprits, but any medication, from aspirin to vaccines, can cause an allergic reaction.*

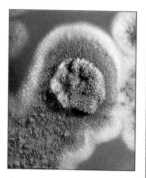

**PENICILLIUM MOLD**
*Commonly found throughout the house, this mold naturally produces penicillin and can cause allergies itself.*

With any form of medication, a doctor weighs the potential risks and benefits before prescribing it. This means that drugs known to be allergic troublemakers are still in common use because they are such powerful elements of the doctor's arsenal against disease. Most important of all are the antibiotics. Penicillins, a major class of antibiotics, are the most widely prescribed drugs in the world.

## ANTIBACTERIALS

The discovery of the antibacterial properties of penicillin is a familiar tale, but antibiotics have been in use for thousands of years. The Chinese have been using moldy soybean curd as a locally applied antibacterial for at least two and a half millennia, and a tradi-

tional British folk treatment for cuts is an old spider web. In all these cases the antibiotic effect derives from mold—or rather from substances produced by mold.

### Penicillins

Of all the antibacterials, penicillins are the most common cause of drug allergies. A study in Boston in 1976 estimated that at least 5 percent of the U.S. population is allergic to the ampicillin form. Typically, penicillin allergy causes an itchy rash, but in extreme cases it can trigger life-threatening anaphylaxis, particularly if the patient has previously had a reaction.

If any sort of reaction occurs, the patient should stop taking the drug immediately, and the doctor will consider prescribing an

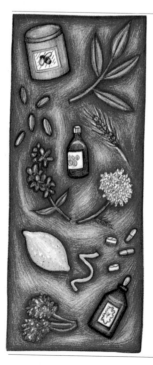

## ANTIBACTERIALS AND ALTERNATIVE REMEDIES

The table below shows the antibacterial drugs that would most often be prescribed for some common conditions, alongside other remedies that you could try. Remember not to disregard your doctor's advice; this list is only a guide.

| CONDITION | MEDICATIONS | OTHER TREATMENTS |
|---|---|---|
| Sore throat (caused by a bacterium) | Penicillins (narrow spectrum) Sulfa drugs | Honey and lemon drink; saltwater gargle; horehound lozenges; gargle of sage or thyme infusion—use every four hours; aspirin gargle (for adults); tea of slippery elm (the inner bark) |
| Chest infections | Penicillins (broad spectrum) Cephalosporins | Honey and lemon drink; warm liniment rub on back, chest, and throat; hot infusion of elderflower, hyssop, or horehound; inhalation of warming aromatic oils, such as eucalyptus |
| Ear infections | Penicillins Cephalosporins | Almond oil drops at body temperature; compresses soaked in yarrow infusion and placed around ear; acupressure to relieve symptoms; hot compress or hot water bottle on ear to relieve pain |
| Urinary infections | Tetracyclines Sulfa drugs | Barley water (simmer barley and lemon peel in water, then add honey); water and baking soda; parsley tea; juniper berry, eucalyptus, and sandalwood oil in a warm bath; cranberry juice as a preventive measure but not a cure |

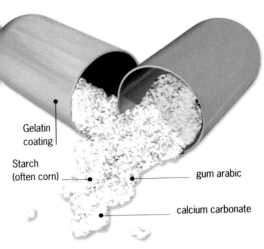

**ADDITIVES IN PILLS**
*Pills and capsules are largely composed of substances like sugar or cornstarch, known as excipients, which are used to carry the active ingredients. Many pills also contain colorings, flavorings, or sugar coatings. Any of these excipients can cause an allergic reaction in a susceptible individual.*

Gelatin coating

Starch (often corn)

gum arabic

calcium carbonate

alternative. If the trigger is subsequently avoided, sensitivity may fade, but no one should resume taking a drug until instructed to do so or, after serious reactions, until it has been shown by means of skin or blood tests conducted in a proper medical setting that the sensitivity has abated.

People who are allergic to penicillin may also be allergic to other antibiotics, in particular the cephalosporins. Several other types of antibiotic, including macrolides such as erythromycin, can, albeit rarely, cause allergy in their own right.

Tetracyclines do not usually trigger acute reactions but extended use as a treatment for acne may cause the buildup of derivative compounds. These are normally inert but can become transformed by sunlight into substances that provoke a reaction known as photodermatitis, in which bright sunlight causes an acute outbreak of hives.

Sulfa drugs, which are used like antibiotics but are created by chemical synthesis rather than derived from molds, can cause rashes and other symptoms. A common group of sulfur-based drugs, the sulfonamides, are frequent culprits.

## Antibiotics in food
Adding antibiotics and other antibacterial agents to animal feed is a widespread practice in the agricultural industry. They are given to livestock, poultry, and fish, and trace amounts can be found in meat, fish,

milk, chicken, and eggs, although at what levels is not always known. Some allergy sufferers are sensitive to even minute quantities of their particular allergen, and there have been reports of reactions that could be due to antibiotic contamination of food.

## OTHER PRESCRIPTION DRUGS
A few other medications are known to produce allergic reactions in some people. These include anti-arrhythmia drugs, antiseizure drugs (for the heart), and allo-purinol, which is prescribed for gout.

## ASPIRIN AND OTHER NSAIDS
A number of pain-relieving drugs can be bought over the counter and taken without medical supervision. In some ways this makes them riskier than antibiotics. Many people—at least 19 percent of adult asthmatics and up to 40 percent of people with nasal polyps (small nodules in the nose) or chronic sinusitis—are sensitive to aspirin, as well as other nonsteroidal anti-inflammatory drugs (NSAIDs), such as ibuprofen. This sensitivity is not considered a true allergy, but typical symptoms include itchiness, hives, runny nose, nasal congestion, watery or swollen eyes, cough, and wheezing.

Aspirin, or salicylic acid, is related to salicylate compounds found in the bark of the willow tree (genus *Salix*) and some other plants. Anyone who is allergic to aspirin should seek advice from a dietitian about avoiding foods that have a high salicylate content, which includes apricots, peppers, and some spices.

## VACCINES
In the past vaccines were made from horse serum or were cultured in eggs. This obviously posed problems for people allergic to horses or eggs. However, the amount of such material in current vaccines is very small and rarely causes trouble. If you are sensitive to horses or eggs, however, make it known before you are given a vaccination. If necessary, the shot can be given in a hospital to be on the safe side.

## THREE REASONS TO AVOID ANTIBIOTICS
Antibiotics are valuable in the fight against infection, but many doctors are growing more cautious about using them.

▶ *Excessive prescribing of antibiotics is leading to the evolution of drug-resistant strains of bacteria. Prescribing fewer drugs may help to slow this development.*

▶ *If your immune system is left to cope with minor infections on its own, you tend to develop stronger immunity, so if the infection recurs, you will be better able to fight it off, unaided by medication.*

▶ *Antibiotics may kill off some of the friendly bacteria in your gut. This makes it easier for unfriendly microbes to invade, causing problems like diarrhea.*

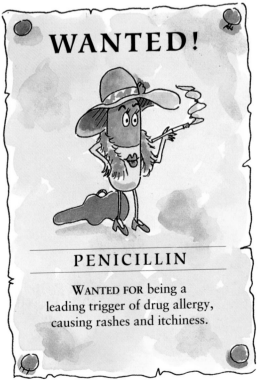

# WANTED!

## PENICILLIN

WANTED FOR being a leading trigger of drug allergy, causing rashes and itchiness.

# The Acupuncturist

*Acupuncture is an ancient Chinese treatment for illness that involves the insertion and manipulation of needles at carefully selected places in the body. It is an effective method of pain relief and is used in China as a surgical anesthetic.*

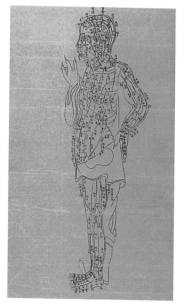

**POWER LINES**
*This ancient Chinese illustration shows just a few of the major acupuncture points, part of a body of knowledge built up over thousands of years.*

Acupuncture can help allergy sufferers in two ways. First, it can be used to treat or relieve allergic symptoms directly, both acute allergic symptoms such as asthma, eczema, and hives, and chronic Type B symptoms, like depression and general feeling of malaise. Second, acupuncture can help relieve pain. In the Western world acupuncture is being used extensively for this purpose. This includes pain from injury, arthritis, premenstrual syndrome, dysmenorrhea (painful periods), nervous tension, migraine, and sciatica. By acting as a replacement for oral pain killers, acupuncture can reduce the need for medication and therefore the risk of adverse side effects and allergic reactions.

### How does it work?

Acupuncturists believe that energy passes through channels in the body, known as meridians, and that this energy can be accessed through carefully mapped points on the skin. Different meridians relate to different organs, so the insertion and manipulation of needles at the relevant points can relieve symptoms in these organs as well as in other, seemingly unrelated, parts of the body. Acupressure involves applying pressure to these same points to achieve similar ends.

Acupuncture and acupressure points along the meridians are labeled according to their position. For instance, point KID 27 is the 27th point on the kidney meridian.

### What qualifications and training does an acupuncturist have?

Training of acupuncturists varies widely across North America. Each of the 50 American states sets its own regulations, and a few have none. Some two dozen states license, certify, or register acupuncturists, which usually means that they have met certain training requirements—

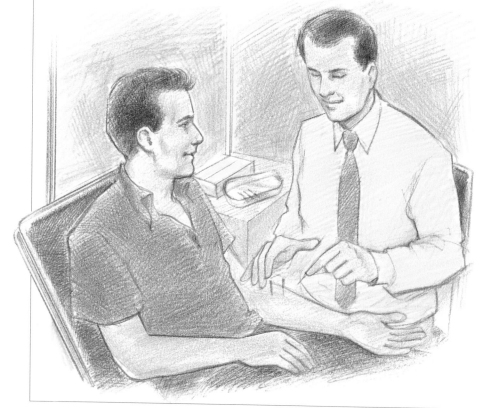

**RELIEF POINTS**
*Acupuncture can provide direct relief from allergy symptoms and can reduce the need for analgesic drugs, thus lowering the chance of allergic reactions.*

usually a three-year course of study—and passed a test developed by the National Commission for the Certification of Acupuncturists. Several states allow only physicians to perform acupuncture, and their qualifications can vary. Some may have trained extensively in China, whereas others may have taken only a brief course in the United States.

Acupuncturists in Canada are not regulated in all the provinces, either, and where they are, in Alberta, for example, such restrictions as prior consultation with a doctor may apply. The University of Alberta in Edmonton and the Acupuncture Foundation of Canada Institute in Toronto offer acupuncture training to physicians and other health care professionals. The Institute of Chinese Medicine and Acupuncture in London, Ontario, has a four-year training program for university graduates with science degrees.

### What evidence is there that acupuncture works?

Some proponents of acupuncture believe that it cannot be assessed by normal scientific methods and they use anecdotal evidence to support their claims. Other acupuncturists have not been so slow off the mark. Described below are just three of a host of studies supporting the use of acupuncture for both pain relief and allergies.

A 1995 study at the Christian Albrechts University in Germany showed that acupuncture provided significantly more relief from migraine than a placebo treatment.

A study of 192 patients published in the *Journal of Traditional Chinese Medicine* in 1990 showed that acupuncture could bring immediate relief to asthma sufferers and was particularly effective for patients with a history of drug allergy.

A controlled study in 1996, at the University Clinic of Physical Therapy and Rehabilitation in the United States, showed that acupuncture on the ear significantly increased the pain threshold of 60 volunteers.

## ACUPRESSURE FOR ALLERGIC RHINITIS

Acupressure works in ways similar to acupuncture but involves finger pressure rather than needles to stimulate pressure points; it can be done anywhere. Acupuncturists recommend placing pressure for two minutes on the following points to relieve the itchiness, watery eyes and nasal passages, and congestion of allergic rhinitis.

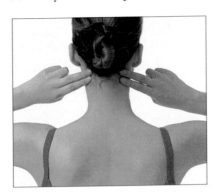

**PRESSURE POINT BL 10**
*This is situated on either side of your spine, about two finger-widths below the base of your skull.*

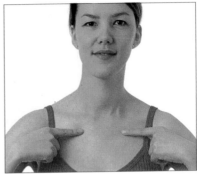

**PRESSURE POINT KID 27**
*This is located just under your collarbones on either side of the breastbone.*

### What do conventional doctors think of this method?

There is a wide spectrum of opinion, ranging from those who reject any medical application for acupuncture to others who firmly believe in its value, in some cases using it regularly in addition to their own conventional treatment methods.

Most doctors fit between these two extremes and are happy for patients to use acupuncture in addition to other treatments. Indeed, among alternative treatments it is one of the most widely accepted, and when performed with proper precautions by a trained practitioner, it is a very safe therapy. Virtually the only risk comes from transfer of infection from inadequately sterilized needles, but most acupuncturists now use disposable needles or meet stringent requirements for sterilizing them.

### Who can benefit from acupuncture?

Skilled practitioners claim that there are few limitations to the range of problems they can treat using acupuncture, but like any other form of therapy it will never be universally successful for all conditions.

## WHAT YOU CAN DO AT HOME

Acupuncture is an activity that you cannot perform on yourself. But acupressure techniques can be done at home and will provide instant relief. Special bands containing magnetized pellets, which help apply constant electromagnetic stimulation to specific points, are available from stores that specialize in health care products. An acupuncturist can advise you if these are appropriate, recommend which points to focus on, and show you how to use acupressure techniques.

**PRESSURE BANDS**
*These bands, which contain magnetized pellets, can be used to steadily stimulate acupressure points on the ankles, wrists, and arms.*

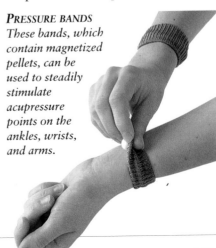

# DRUGS AND NATURAL ALTERNATIVES

*Natural remedies may provoke fewer allergic reactions than synthetic or highly processed drugs, but the only sure way of avoiding a reaction is to reduce your need for medication.*

**WEIGHING YOUR NEED FOR DRUGS**
*A decision to use medication is based on an assessment of the benefits it might provide versus the risk it entails. Doctors and patients alike must weigh their options before deciding.*

There are three cornerstones to reducing the likelihood of developing an allergic reaction to drugs. The first is to reassess your need for medication. Do you really need a pill, or will your problem subside soon of its own accord? The second is to substitute a natural remedy for a synthetic drug. Third, and most important, is to reduce your need for medication by improving your mental and physical well-being, so that you don't need to take drugs in the first place.

### RESTRICT YOUR DRUG USE

Any decision to take drugs should be based on necessity rather than convenience. Before reaching for an aspirin, ask yourself a few questions. Do you have an intense pain or simply a passing irritation? Is your problem self-limiting—in other words, will it go away on its own without intervention? Can you effectively ignore it and get on with other activities? Are your symptoms telling you something you should not ignore? For instance, recurring headaches might indicate that you should look for the underlying cause, rather than using pain relievers.

Obviously, there is a scale of severity. At one extreme, no one would seek to deny pain-relieving drugs to cancer sufferers, but at the other end of the scale, many people are guilty of overreliance on painkillers and other drugs to cope with minor discomforts. you can learn to weigh your need for medication against the possible risks and side effects it may produce.

### BASIC PRECAUTIONS WITH DRUGS

You should use prescription drugs only for the condition for which they were prescribed and never give your prescriptions to others. Diagnosis is difficult enough even with proper medical training. If you attempt to diagnose yourself or others, you might miss important clues to a dangerous disorder. Self-medicating then compounds the mistake. Not only do you risk taking the wrong drug, but there may be subtleties of which you are not aware. Because of issues like the timing of doses and the dangers of interactions with other drugs the prescription of drugs requires expert training.

Try to minimize your use of drugs in general. They should be a last, not a first, resort. Become fit and healthy enough to prevent illness and look for other ways to control simple problems.

Always follow instructions. The precise timing of your dose may be crucial: some must be taken only with food or they will not be properly absorbed. For others the

### DRUGS DON'T AGE WELL

Never use a drug after the expiration date on the label. The substances that make up a drug may be volatile or reactive, and their effectiveness depends on their exact composition. Like all organic substances, of which most pharmaceuticals are composed, they will degrade and break down with time. Some medications will merely become inactive, but others— for example, the topical antibiotic tetracycline that is often prescribed for people with dermatitis—become toxic with increased age. This applies to both prescription and over-the-counter medicines.

*Practical Steps for*

# Stress Relief

*Your state of mind can have an enormous influence on your physical health, including the strength of your immune system, your threshold for pain, and your sensitivity to allergens. Reducing your stress levels can improve your overall health.*

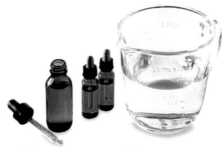

To better control the stress in your life and improve your health as a result, it will help to take a look at a number of lifestyle factors.

## Planning

Prioritizing your time, learning to delegate, and being prepared will help you achieve your goals in the time allotted for them. Make a plan for the week ahead and then keep a diary of what you achieve. Compare the two and identify what went right and where problems arose.

### Natural stress relief remedies

Exercise can relieve stress and make you more resistant to illness. Activities like t'ai chi and yoga can help you become fit and develop relaxation skills. You can even use stretching and flexibility exercises to combat pain directly without drugs.

Bach remedies, essences of flowering plants available in health food and natural remedy stores, are a safe means of counteracting stress and will not interfere with any medication you are taking.

### CONCOCT YOUR OWN

*You can make your own Bach remedies for stressful situations by diluting and mixing 2 drops each of any of the plants listed below in a 30 ml (2 oz) dropper bottle filled with mineral water.*

*Elm is a good remedy to use when you are feeling overwhelmed or unable to cope. Walnut helps in adapting to new environments and situations. Impatiens can help you feel better when you can't keep up with a hectic schedule.*

## STRETCHES TO EASE TENSION

Stress and backache often go together, particularly in the office. Try the simple exercise shown here to help relieve tension and backache. Do not try this if you have severe back, muscle, or joint problems. See a doctor, osteopath, or physiotherapist.

**Keep** your back straight and your head facing forward.

### LOOK UP
*Holding the rest of your body in a stable position, stretch your raised arm by reaching as high as you can. Now turn your head slowly until you are looking up the length of your arm. Straighten up slowly, returning to the start position, and repeat on the other side.*

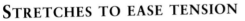

### SPREAD YOUR ARMS
*Stretch your arms out horizontally. Your feet should be shoulder-width apart.*

**Stand** with legs straight and knees relaxed, not locked.

### LEAN TO THE SIDE
*Keeping your face forward, lean over to one side, spreading your arms in a straight line so that one points up while the other points down. Try not to twist your body; keep it in line with your hips to avoid putting your back under pressure.*

**Reach** down along your leg, stretching as far as you can go without lowering your shoulder. The movement should come from your waist.

**CLEAN LIVING**
*A healthy lifestyle, with exercise, good diet, and limited stress, is the best protection against ill health of all kinds, allergies included.*

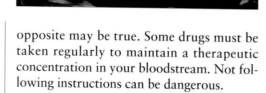

**MEDICINE MAN**
*Shamans, witch doctors, and medicine men, like the one pictured below, rely overwhelmingly on natural remedies. These may provoke fewer allergic reactions than Western drugs, but there are no safeguards against the inclusion of toxic ingredients in them. Each approach has its disadvantages.*

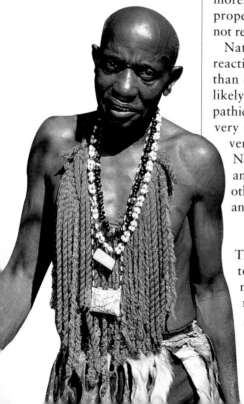

opposite may be true. Some drugs must be taken regularly to maintain a therapeutic concentration in your bloodstream. Not following instructions can be dangerous.

### NATURAL REMEDIES

The availability of drugs for managing pain, infections, and other health problems is a relatively recent phenomenon. For most of human history we have relied on the sort of techniques that the majority of the world's population still relies upon—natural remedies prepared mainly from plants. These remedies often depend on potent ingredients that are much like those of modern pharmaceuticals, many of which are derived or developed from plant sources themselves.

This means that natural remedies should be approached with as much caution as conventional medicines—in some cases with more, because they may not have been properly tested, and their manufacture is not regulated to consistent standards.

Natural remedies can produce allergic reactions, but in general they are milder than conventional medicines and are less likely to cause severe side effects. Homeopathic remedies in particular, are generally very safe because they involve the use of very low concentrations of substances. Nonetheless, you should always consult an herbalist, homeopath, naturopath, or other qualified practitioner before using any natural remedies.

### A HEALTHY LIFESTYLE

The best way to avoid using drugs is not to need them. The vast majority of minor complaints and many of the major ones are eminently preventable. A healthy, balanced diet, adequate exercise, moderate drinking, not smoking, and reducing stress levels make up the most effective preventive treatment you can find anywhere.

Poor diet and nutritional deficiencies are implicated in many allergic conditions—one example is magnesium deficiency in asthma (see page 74)—and in general, physical and mental health. Lack of exercise can make you unfit and overweight, major risk factors for many types of disease. Exercise is an excellent way to reduce stress.

Alcohol and smoking are also implicated in many allergic illnesses and related conditions, both directly and indirectly. Alcohol and some of the elements of cigarette smoke can act as allergens or irritants themselves, exacerbating or causing allergic conditions such as asthma. Indirectly, they can impair general health and the proper functioning of the immune system.

Although allergic individuals need to identify and avoid the substances that trigger their symptoms, the benefits of a healthy lifestyle could make a radical difference to the frequency and severity of these health problems. In fact, if you follow a healthy lifestyle, you can reduce the incidence in your life of migraine and other headaches, aches, colds, stomach upsets, influenza, and infections of all kinds.

### NATURAL REMEDIES FOR PAIN RELIEF

By cutting down on your use of drugs you can reduce the chances of developing an allergic reaction. One way of doing this is to treat mild illnesses with natural remedies.

Camphor oil and chamomile tea can help ease rheumatic pain. Applying a poultice of feverfew or ingesting the leaves reduces the severity of migraine, gargling with sage tea can help ease throat pain, and drinking peppermint tea may relieve indigestion.

Hydrotherapy can be a simple and effective home remedy for many types of pain. Hot and cold compresses, applied alternately for 20 to 30 minutes (3 minutes hot, 1 minute cold), can help to relieve many muscular and joint pains. The pain of a sore throat can also be relieved with a cold compress.

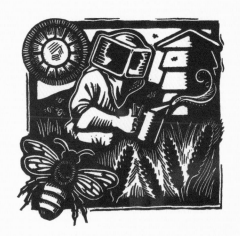

# CHAPTER 7

# OTHER ALLERGIES

*Inhalant, food, drug, and contact allergies account for the vast majority of allergic reactions, but there are many others. Some of them may afflict relatively few people across the country, but this makes them no less serious. In rare cases these conditions can cause fatal anaphylaxis.*

# INSECT ALLERGIES

*It is well known that wasp and bee stings can cause severe reactions, even fatal anaphylaxis. Other insects have also brought on anaphylaxis, but such incidences are rare.*

## Fear of flying things

Only an unlucky few are in serious danger from a bee or wasp sting, and thanks to the treatment available, stings cause very few deaths each year. In the United States, for instance, one person in 6 million dies from an insect sting each year. If you are are allergic to wasp or bee stings, you should carry your own adrenaline kit (see page 128) when you travel, along with a letter signed by your doctor explaining why you need it.

Reactions to insect bites and stings can take several forms. Most people suffer a mild local response after being stung by a wasp or bee or bitten by a mosquito or flea. The sting or bite causes a small, inflamed swelling accompanied by a hot, throbbing pain or itching, and the symptoms generally clear up within a day or two.

Someone is said to be allergic when a bite or sting produces an inappropriately severe reaction. In such a person the immune system overreacts, causing the release of histamine and other inflammatory agents. If this happens locally, it results in a larger than usual swelling and more intense itching.

If swellings appear at sites other than the bite or sting, this is a systemic reaction, which can be dangerous and even lead to anaphylactic shock. Fortunately deaths from anaphylaxis caused by insect stings are rare. Their annual incidence is about 40 in the United States. That the death rate is so low can be attributed mainly to susceptible people carrying the medications they need and getting prompt medical attention. (Even after the danger has passed, someone who has suffered anaphylaxis should see a doctor.)

### INSECTS THAT CAUSE ALLERGIES

Insects from the Hymenoptera order—which includes bees, wasps, and ants—are the main cause of sting allergies. The bee is potentially the most dangerous because it leaves its stinger in the victim's skin and the venom sac continues to pump in poison. However, stings from bees are quite rare because most are not very aggressive. (The exception is the Aftrican killer bee, which in recent years has mated with honeybees in North America. When excited, these hybrid bees may attack in great numbers.)

Stings from wasps and hornets are much more common because of their more aggressive nature and habits. For instance, wasps are attracted to sweet foods and meat and thus are drawn to places where people eat; stings are common under such circumstances.

### LOCAL AND SYSTEMIC REACTIONS

In someone who is not allergic, the bite or venom causes a localized reaction with a swelling of no more than 2 centimeters (about ¾ inch) in diameter. In some people the swelling may reach 10 centimeters (4 inches) in diameter and last for more than 24 hours. A very small percentage of victims suffer a systemic reaction.

### Systemic reactions

A systemic reaction is a fairly immediate, generalized response to a sting or bite. Anaphylaxis is the technical term for all systemic reactions, but it is used most often to mean a very severe one. Mild systemic reac-

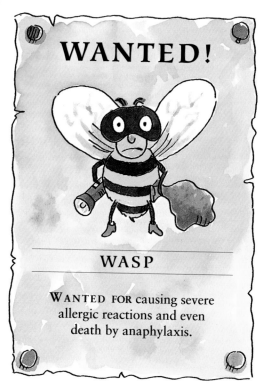

**WANTED!**

**WASP**

**WANTED FOR** causing severe allergic reactions and even death by anaphylaxis.

## ALLERGENIC INSECTS

The insect order that causes the most allergy problems is Hymenoptera. There are three insect families in this group: Apidae (colloquially called Apids)—honeybees, and bumblebees; Vespidae (Vespids)—wasps and hornets; and Formicidae, which includes the fire ant.

Other insects whose bites or stings have been known to cause allergic reactions include bedbugs, fleas, mites, ticks, horseflies, midges, mosquitoes, and spiders, including those that are not poisonous to humans. The insects below are not shown to scale.

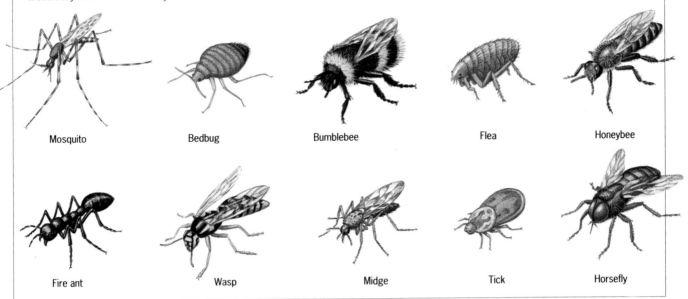

Mosquito    Bedbug    Bumblebee    Flea    Honeybee

Fire ant    Wasp    Midge    Tick    Horsefly

tions are characterized by widespread itching, swollen eyes, and diarrhea. Severe anaphylaxis can cause breathing difficulties and a dangerous drop in blood pressure; it is a medical emergency. Anaphylaxis responds well to prompt administration of epinephrine (adrenaline) and antihistamines; patients at risk should carry a kit containing these (see page 128) when there is a chance of being stung. Mild anaphylaxis tends to become worse on subsequent encounters with an allergenic insect; anyone who has experienced hives or angioedema on at least one occasion should probably carry epinephrine.

### How do you know if you are at risk?

A previous reaction to a sting or bite is the biggest risk factor for a serious allergic reaction. If you have never had a severe reaction, you probably do not need to worry. However, anaphylaxis is unpredictable, and some individuals who die from it may have had no previous history of sting allergy. There is a blood test that can check for sensitivity to Hymenoptera venom, but a negative result does not totally exclude the possibility of a reaction; some people who test positive have previously shown no reaction to stings. If you should be positive on

testing, consider a course of venom immunotherapy, which will reduce the potential for severe reactions.

Being stung frequently can increase the likelihood of developing hypersensitivity, but if there are long intervals between stings, a reaction may become less likely. This is because the level of IgE (the immunoglobin that causes an allergic response to insect stings) specific to that insect's venom will often diminish over time.

### What if you are stung?

Bee stings in particular are more dangerous because bees impart a greater dose of venom than wasps and hornets (see page 124). Currently, the best advice to anyone who has previously suffered a systemic reaction to stings is to carry epinephrine. If stung, administer the medication immediately and call for emergency medical help.

### OTHER INSECTS THAT CAUSE ALLERGIC REACTIONS

Mosquito bites can cause swelling and irritation at the site of the bite, and these can last for several days. Such reactions are more common in children and are hardly ever serious. In some parts of the world,

# Insect Allergies

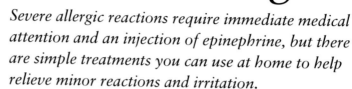

*Severe allergic reactions require immediate medical attention and an injection of epinephrine, but there are simple treatments you can use at home to help relieve minor reactions and irritation.*

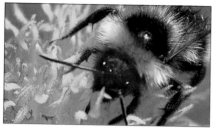

**HONEYBEE**
*The honeybee,* Apis mellifera, *is found throughout North America. It is one of many species of bee with a barbed sting.*

All stings cause pain, itching, and swelling at the site of the sting. If a systemic reaction occurs, it usually starts within half an hour. When a bee stinger is left in the skin, it should be scraped away with a knife blade, fingernail, credit card, or similar object. Do not use tweezers because squeezing the venom sac may force more venom into the body.

## TREATING LOCAL IRRITATION

If an insect bite or sting produces only local irritation, swelling, and pain, you can take acetaminophen to relieve the pain and an antihistamine tablet to relieve irritation. Antihistamine cream may also help.

Time-honored natural remedies for soothing bites and stings include a paste of baking soda (see below); a poultice made with the leaves of the plantain (*Plantago lanceolata*), a weed that grows all over North America; and aloe vera gel, prefer-

ably a scoop from a fresh leaf rather than a commercial preparation.

For bee or wasp stings homeopaths often prescribe one tablet of *Apis mel* every 15 minutes for an hour or so, depending on the severity of the sting. Also used for stings is *Ledum,* one full tablet every 10 to 15 minutes for the first hour, then one tablet every three hours until the pain subsides. If there is any sign of a more serious reaction, get medical help right away.

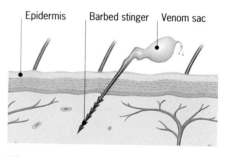

Epidermis    Barbed stinger    Venom sac

**HOW A STING WORKS**
*A barbed stinger is left in the skin of a victim, along with the venom sac, which continues to pump poison.*

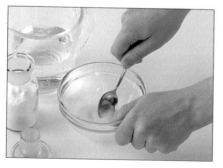

**BEE STINGS**
*For bee stings or insect bites a soothing treatment is a paste of water and baking soda (sodium bicarbonate) applied to the area of the sting. A mouthwash of baking soda (one teaspoon in a glass of water) makes a quick, soothing remedy for a bee sting to the mouth, but as a precaution, you should follow up with a visit to a doctor.*

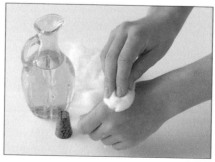

**WASP STINGS**
*For wasp stings you can use plain cider vinegar. (Do not confuse this treatment with baking soda for a bee sting.) After applying treatment for either a wasp or bee sting, wrap a bag of ice in a towel and hold it over the site of the sting. An alternative folk remedy is to apply a slice of raw onion to the sting, holding it in place with cotton bandage or scarf.*

### EPINEPHRINE

If you know that you will have a systemic reaction to a sting, you should carry epinephrine (adrenaline) with you at all times when a sting might occur. If anaphylaxis starts, you must be given the epinephrine—as an injection in the outer side of the thigh or a spray to the inside of the mouth—and antihistamines right away then go to an emergency medical center, in case you need more intervention. If you are not carrying adrenaline, it is essential that you seek medical help immediately.

however, mosquitoes carry malarial parasites, which can cause allergic reactions in addition to malaria. Certain antihistamines, such as cetirizine (Zyrtec), can suppress the allergic symptoms if taken immediately after a bite or in anticipation of being bitten.

Other biting insects that usually cause only moderate reactions in allergic individuals can trigger anaphylaxis in rare cases. These include horse, deer, and blackflies, midges, fleas, ticks, lice, and some spiders. Bedbugs (*Cimex* species) can cause large, raised wheals in rare cases. These can be treated with the methods described on the opposite page. Try not to scratch an insect bite because this will increase the irritation.

A particular problem with ticks is that they bury their mouth parts in the skin when they bite. If a tick is not removed with care, the mouthparts can be left behind and cause irritation and even infection. Applying nail polish to the exposed body of the tick should cause it to loosen its grip, making it easier to remove safely. (Watch out for a circular rash surrounding a tick bite. It could indicate an infection with Lyme disease, a serious illness that requires immediate treatment with antibiotics.)

## AVOIDING BITES AND STINGS

Certain scents and clothing attract stinging insects and others repel them. There are also certain places where insects are more likely to congregate and particular situations in which they are more likely to become aggressive. The chart below describes some of the most common risk factors and what to do about them.

### If you are attacked

If you spot a swarm of bees, keep well away and notify a local beekeeper or a pest control company. Do not panic: swarms are usually less aggressive than single bees because they have eaten all the honey they can carry, which makes them relatively docile. Try to move slowly and without any sudden movements until you are a safe distance away. If you are attacked, cover your head with your arms or some clothing; bees and wasps go instinctively for the dark patches on faces—the mouth, eyes, nostrils, and ears.

If you come across a wasp nest in the deck or eaves of your home, move slowly away. You can ignore the nest and get rid of it after it is abandoned. If it poses problems, ask a pest control company to remove it.

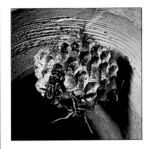

***WASP NEST***
*Common spots for wasp nests are under the eaves of houses and in trees, including old tree trunks. Generally wasps in temperate areas have active nests only during the spring, summer, and fall. During the winter, the queen hibernates and the other wasps die off.*

## PREVENTING INSECT BITES AND STINGS

As with any allergy, prevention is the most effective approach, so avoiding insect bites and stings in the first place is the best way to spare yourself a nasty reaction. The chart below describes some of the factors and situations that can attract or aggravate insects, especially wasps, hornets, and bees, and offers tips and strategies to help you minimize the risk of being stung or bitten.

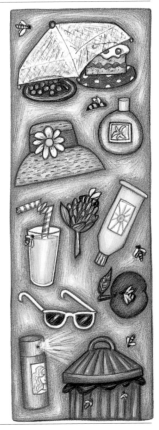

| RISK FACTOR | DO'S AND DON'TS |
|---|---|
| Scents | Perfumes, hairsprays, strongly scented sun creams, and shampoos—all attract wasps and other vespids. They are also attracted to sweat and the carbon dioxide in a person's breath, so take care when exercising outside. |
| Movements | Avoid sudden movements when approached by a stinging insect. |
| Being inside | Keep windows shut or covered with screens and food and garbage cans covered. |
| Being outside | Avoid orchards with fallen ripe fruit because these attract wasps. Do not disturb fallen tree trunks because wasps and bees are likely to nest in these. Bees are attracted to clover in the grass, and they also nest in the ground. Keep food covered when eating outside and avoid places where animals are fed. |
| Clothing | Avoid flapping or brightly colored clothing: neutral-colored, green, or brown clothes are best.<br>Stay covered up while gardening, with long pants and long-sleeved shirts.<br>Wear a hat and gloves for extra protection.<br>Wear gloves and a helmet when riding a motorbike. When riding a bicycle try to keep your mouth shut, and wear sunglasses. Do not walk barefoot outside. |

# UNUSUAL ALLERGIES

*Some unusual skin allergies have been recorded. They are reactions to substances that are important or even vital to life, and as varied as water, sunlight, and even other people.*

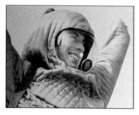

***STAYING INSIDE***
*A few people develop so many sensitivities that they stay well only in special allergen-free environments, as in the 1977 TV film,* The Boy in the Plastic Bubble. *It starred John Travolta, pictured here in an environmental isolation suit. The allergies and sensitivities themselves may not be unusual, but having so many of them is, fortunately, rare.*

In theory, you can become allergic to just about anything, and there are unusual allergies that can be debilitating and even life-threatening. For instance, some individuals develop symptoms when they are with certain people, most often in response to some perfume, soap, or pet dander on the other person's body. Allergies to people themselves are rare but can be caused by skin particles, hair, or fluid. Reactions are more likely to occur in a person who is already suffering from eczema.

Some women are allergic to seminal fluid; they break out in hives or even, very rarely, experience anaphylaxis. Reactions can be avoided if the male withdraws before ejaculation or uses a condom. Some men react to feminine hygiene sprays used by their partner prior to intercourse.

Both partners can develop skin reactions to propylene glycol, an ingredient of some lubricating agents. Reactions to the latex in a rubber diaphragm or condom sheath may occur in the vulva, vagina, or penis. Polyurethane condoms are available for those who are allergic to rubber, but some people are sensitive to these as well.

Vulval inflammation can also be caused by douches, feminine hygiene sprays, and skin medications. Allergic reactions may result from vaginal spermicides, hair-removing agents, soaps, bubble baths, some sanitary pads, and the residues of chemicals left on the hands.

## TEMPERATURE SENSITIVITY

In rare circumstances sunlight can induce a rapid onset of hives. The electromagnetic radiation in the sun's rays triggers the mast cells in the skin to discharge their inflammatory contents, including histamine.

Cold skin from very low air temperatures or contact with ice or snow can also cause hives. If the whole body is exposed, for instance, by a fall into icy water, a state similar to that of anaphylactic shock could occur, which is thought to be due to excess histamine production. In such a case, immediate medical attention is needed.

## WATER SENSITIVITY

Certain chemicals in tap water can cause allergic reactions. Chlorine in swimming pools can be a problem, too; even the lesser concentrations in tap water sometimes cause reactions. It may be necessary to use filtered or bottled water for drinking and washing.

In a vary rare condition called aquagenic urticaria, skin develops hives when exposed to any water: tap, distilled, even the person's own sweat or tears. This reaction is caused by the chemical acetylcholine, which is released when water touches skin. The drug scopolamine is used to treat the condition.

---

### FILTERING WATER

People sensitive to water contaminants should use filtered water for drinking and washing. A jug filter may be adequate, but a filter installed in the water system is usually more effective and convenient.

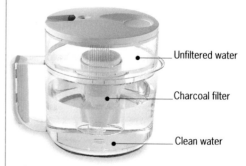

Unfiltered water

Charcoal filter

Clean water

***ALLERGY-FREE WATER***
*A jug filter should remove contaminants such as chlorine, nitrates, pesticides, and lead, and may even soften hard water.*

# ANAPHYLAXIS

*The sudden onset of severe allergic symptoms—intense itchiness, swelling of the face, racing pulse, and difficulty breathing— signals an anaphylactic response. This is a medical emergency.*

People most at risk for severe anaphylaxis (anaphylactic, or septic, shock) are those who have had an intense reaction to an allergen before. But anyone can suffer an attack, even someone who has not had previous symptoms to warn him. How can you recognize the danger signs if you've never had a reaction before?

### SYMPTOMS

The first symptom is often a foreboding that all is not well. This is followed—particularly if a food is the cause—by immediate burning, irritation, or itching of the lips, mouth, and throat. Other signs are swelling of the mouth, face, tongue, and throat, causing difficulty in swallowing or speaking; swelling of the airways and consequent breathing problems; a rash or hives; and stomach problems, like nausea or cramps. Blood pressure often drops dramatically, followed by weakness and unconsciousness.

In children the first sign is often a change in the color of their skin, like blotchiness on the chest, or purple fingers, which, after blanching (going pale) then being squeezed, do not recover their color quickly.

Death can result, either from suffocation because the throat is blocked by swelling or from heart failure because of the fall in blood pressure. It should be stressed that these are rare manifestations of an untreated severe reaction. Less severe cases may recover spontaneously, while prompt treatment ensures recovery for others.

### COMMON TRIGGERS

Penicillin is the most common trigger of anaphylaxis, followed by such foods as milk, peanuts, fish, shellfish, or eggs, then wasp and bee stings. Other causes include vaccines, immunotherapy, blood transfusions, natural latex, and in some cases, exercise. Although anaphylaxis is unpredictable, it is more likely to occur in patients who have had severe urticaria in the past. Other risk factors include older age, asthma, especially in children, and taking beta-blockers (prescribed for heart problems and other conditions). Also, people who are atopic—that is, those who have a generally high level of IgE and are thus highly sensitive to allergenic substances—may be at slightly greater risk than most individuals.

### Exercise-induced anaphylaxis

In rare cases anaphylaxis may be provoked by exercise. Sometimes this happens only with a combination of exercise and the eating of a specific food a few hours beforehand. In such cases, neither factor precipitates an attack on its own. Other things that may contribute to the onset of exercise-induced anaphylaxis are working out in an extremely hot or cold environment or in

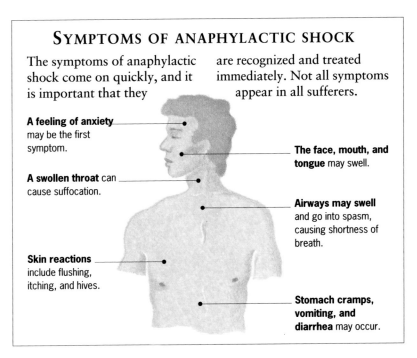

**TRIGGER FOODS**
*Anaphylactic reactions to food are rare, but some foods are known to head the list of anaphylactic triggers. Peanuts are at the top, and tree nuts also rank high.*

## SYMPTOMS OF ANAPHYLACTIC SHOCK

The symptoms of anaphylactic shock come on quickly, and it is important that they are recognized and treated immediately. Not all symptoms appear in all sufferers.

**A feeling of anxiety** may be the first symptom.

**A swollen throat** can cause suffocation.

**Skin reactions** include flushing, itching, and hives.

**The face, mouth, and tongue** may swell.

**Airways may swell** and go into spasm, causing shortness of breath.

**Stomach cramps, vomiting, and diarrhea** may occur.

## TREATING ANAPHYLAXIS

In treating anaphylaxis, act quickly—dial 911, then administer epinephrine and antihistamines. The patient should be laid down, feet elevated, unless he is having breathing difficulties. If breathing or heartbeat stops, perform CPR.

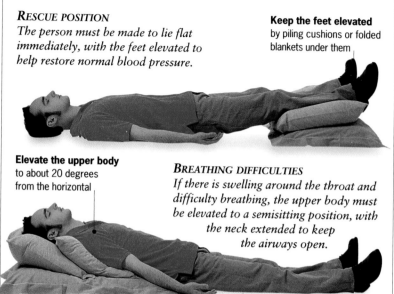

*RESCUE POSITION*
*The person must be made to lie flat immediately, with the feet elevated to help restore normal blood pressure.*

**Keep the feet elevated** by piling cushions or folded blankets under them

**Elevate the upper body** to about 20 degrees from the horizontal

*BREATHING DIFFICULTIES*
*If there is swelling around the throat and difficulty breathing, the upper body must be elevated to a semisitting position, with the neck extended to keep the airways open.*

high humidity, exercising while menstruating, ingesting a drug (aspirin, for instance) before exercise, and a hot shower after exercise.

### Vaccine anaphylaxis

Anaphylactic reactions to vaccines are also rare and unpredictable and may occur in people who have no known risk factors. During the 1994 measles and rubella immunization campaign in the United Kingdom, 81 cases of anaphylaxis were reported out of about 8 million children immunized, and there were no deaths. Doctors keep epinephrine on hand when giving immunizations.

### Latex anaphylaxis

A small but increasing number of people are extremely allergic to the latex in natural rubber. Those particularly at risk are people who work in the rubber industry and medical personnel who use rubber gloves. Anyone who undergoes many surgical procedures can also be in danger because more of the allergen can be readily absorbed during surgery. Other sources of latex include pacifiers, rubber toys and balloons, condoms, diaphrams, and rubber bands.

Anyone who has suffered severe latex allergy must warn a doctor or dentist before undergoing any examination or procedure, in case the practitioner uses latex gloves. Nonlatex alternatives, which include vinyl and synthetic latex, are available.

### TREATMENT

Fast treatment is essential. At the onset of an anaphylactic reaction, the sufferer should be made to lie down and, most important, be given epinephrine (adrenaline). People who know they are susceptible to anaphylactic shock should always carry their own adrenaline in a preloaded syringe for self-injection or as a spray. The adrenaline should be injected in the side of the leg.

Some patients are prescribed an adrenaline inhaler instead. In an emergency these are used to spray the inside of the cheek, using at least 20 sprays for an adult. This form of medication is easier and less intimidating than self-injection. Sufferers should also carry antihistamine and use it in emergencies, provided they can swallow.

An emergency adrenaline shot is only the first step in the treatment of anaphylaxis. Further treatment with more adrenaline and other drugs is often essential. Anyone who has suffered an anaphylactic episode should seek medical attention, even if they appear to be recovering. Occasionally, patients suffer a relapse, sometimes even the next day, and they require further treatment.

### PRECAUTIONS

People who know they are susceptible to anaphylaxis should carry a warning card or wear a pendant with the details of their allergy. They should also carry a prescribed emergency kit at all times. Trainer kits are available that teach the patient and relatives how to use the medications. A child's teacher should be vigilant; children may be offered allergenic foods by their friends without realizing the danger. Everyone should know where to find the epinephrine and how to give it in an emergency.

> **WARNING**
> *Epinephrine may be dangerous for people with heart disease. For children, a teacher or school nurse must be trained to recognize the symptoms of anaphylaxis and how to give the epinephrine.*

# CHAPTER 8

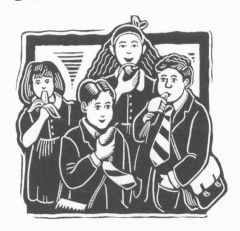

# CHILDREN AND ALLERGY

*From persistent coughs and sleepless
nights to behavioral disorders and educational
underachievement, the problems caused by
allergies can make a child's life—and that of the
parents—very difficult. If doctors and parents
know what to look for and how to deal with it,
they can make a huge difference to a child's
health, mental well-being, and future.*

# PREVENTION OF ALLERGIES

*Taking special care from the time you become pregnant until your baby is two years old can help to avoid years of caring for a child with allergies.*

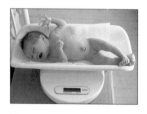

***BIRTH WEIGHT AND ALLERGY***
*Good nutrition for a mother increases the chance that her baby will grow to a good size and that the pregnancy will continue to full term. There is evidence of an association between low birth weight and the development of asthma and possibly other allergies as well.*

It is known that a tendency to develop allergies runs in families. Research indicates that this tendency has a complex pattern of inheritance and there is little likelihood of screening tests for susceptibility to allergies being developed in the near future.

To reduce the chance of having a baby prone to allergies, start planning at least three months before you hope to become pregnant. There is growing evidence that a woman's nutrition, environment, and lifestyle during this time can influence the later development of allergies in her child.

## DIETARY FACTORS

It is essential that a woman who wants to conceive pay close attention to her nutrition, starting before conception and continuing until the end of breast feeding. During this period she needs more of certain nutrients than usual. Dietary nutrients, particularly zinc, selenium, magnesium, and certain vitamins, mainly the B group, have a major effect on the development and proper functioning of the immune system. A well-balanced diet that includes ample fruits, vegetables, and whole grains should provide them. However, it might be wise to consult a nutritionist and consider taking a supplement specially designed by experts for use during pregnancy. It is important to get good advice because high-dose supplements can be especially harmful to a fetus.

This dietary advice does not apply only to mothers; a man's sperm count and quality may be adversely affected by poor nutrition. A few months of nutritional therapy may be needed to correct any problems.

## NUTRITION DURING PREGNANCY

Throughout pregnancy and while breastfeeding a mother should have a varied diet, avoiding large amounts of any one food, especially dairy products. Evidence shows that foreign proteins, such as the casein in cow's milk, can cross the placenta from the bloodstream of a mother to a fetus and can get into breast milk.

***BABY FOOD***
*Eat a variety of healthful foods, avoiding the main food allergy triggers.*

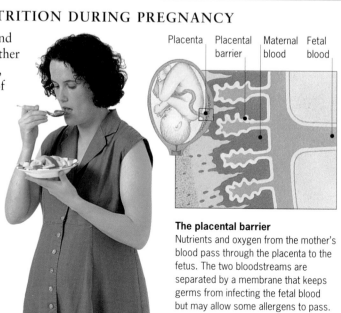

**The placental barrier**
Nutrients and oxygen from the mother's blood pass through the placenta to the fetus. The two bloodstreams are separated by a membrane that keeps germs from infecting the fetal blood but may allow some allergens to pass.

## Mother-child transfer of allergens

The developing immune system in a fetus and a baby under three months old is still learning to distinguish between its own tissue, which it needs to tolerate, and foreign material, which it must reject. During this time the immune system is particularly vulnerable to high levels of foreign proteins, which can disturb and interfere with this learning process. They can cause an infant's immune system to become hypersensitive—the condition known as atopy.

For reasons that are not entirely clear, this response can occur with any foreign protein, but is particularly likely to happen with pollen or dust and also with milk, if it forms a large part of the mother's diet.

## Breast versus bottle feeding

A baby's intestines have a role in determining whether the child develops allergies. For at least three months after birth a baby's gut continues to develop. Breast milk helps the gut mature and reduces the absorption of proteins that might lead to allergies. Ideally it should be the sole source of nutrition, with weaning delayed until at least four months and preferably not until one year.

Many mothers give up breast feeding needlessly. This is sometimes because of the growth and behavior pattern of breast-fed babies. They often take more, but shorter, feeds than bottle-fed babies and may not gain weight as rapidly in the first few months. These features can cause anxiety that the baby is not being satisfied by the breast milk. Get the advice of a pediatrician, midwife, or breast-feeding support group to better understand what is a normal pattern of feeding for a breast-fed baby.

When a baby is bottle fed entirely, or a breast-fed baby is given an occasional supplementary feeding with a bottle, a protein hydrolysate formula should be chosen. This is a partially digested protein formula that is less likely to trigger allergy than milk.

Solid foods, such as fruits, vegetables, and rice, can be introduced—one at a time—after six months, according to the baby's appetite, but the most common allergy triggers should be avoided. After one year of age, milk, wheat, corn, soy products, and citrus fruits can be added, and at two years, eggs and fish. Peanuts should not be offered until age three. Any food that causes a reaction should be discontinued.

### LIFESTYLE FACTORS

Stress is known to affect the body's immune responses, including allergic reactions. It also increases the risk of problems in pregnancy that may lead to low birth weight. Fetuses and babies are able to perceive stress in their environment and may react adversely.

Ideally a mother should be as relaxed as possible throughout pregnancy and during a baby's first year of life. This is a difficult demand to meet because pregnancy, childbirth, and caring for an infant can all cause considerable stress. Reducing stress levels involves planning ahead carefully, and perhaps using some relaxation techniques, such as yoga, aromatherapy, or t'ai chi.

## Smoking

Tobacco smoke greatly increases the risk of asthma in infancy, as well as the likelihood of premature birth and low birth weight. Evidence from a 1978 American study of more than 2,000 patients and from a 1988 Swedish study, published in the *Archives of Diseases in Childhood*, shows that tobacco smoke helps switch on the allergy system.

### ENVIRONMENTAL FACTORS

Heavy exposure to certain products in the atmosphere plays a major role in setting the immune system on the path to allergy. Research particularly implicates high levels of infant exposure to house dust mites, molds, and animal dander (flakes of skin).

Protective measures for children are essentially the same as those for adults (see Chapter 3). A well-ventilated home, kept at an even temperature of 18°–21°C (65°–70°F), with bare floors, washable rugs and curtains, no humid spots, and a minimum of synthetic fabrics, provides a low-allergen environment, keeping dust mites, molds, and chemicals to a minimum. One way to keep a child's blankets and cuddly toys free of dust mites without using toxic antimite chemicals is to wash them regularly in water that is at least 54°C (130°F).

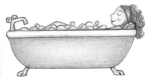

*RELAXING AROMAS*
*Aromatherapy oils added to bath water can be an aid to relaxation, but some oils should be avoided by pregnant women—in particular sage, basil, myrrh, thyme, and marjoram. Lavender oil is safe and relaxing.*

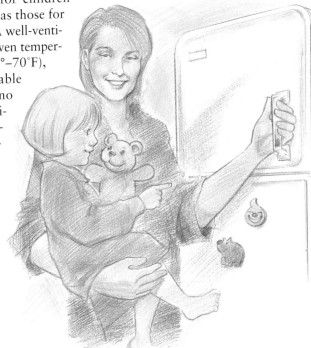

*THE BIG CHILL*
*You can keep down the dust mite population of your child's soft toys with a 12-hour spell in the freezer every two weeks.*

# MANAGING YOUR CHILD'S ALLERGY

*Successfully identifying and managing a child's allergy involves striking a delicate balance between changing and restricting the child's environment and minimizing his or her distress.*

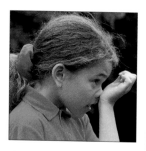

***ALLERGIC SALUTE***
*Allergic rhinitis can cause a persistently itchy, blocked, or runny nose. Children whose noses are constantly dripping develop a habitual response, known as an allergic salute. They push up the end of the nose to wipe away mucus and relieve itchiness.*

How can you tell if your child's illness or discomfort is due to an allergic reaction? How do you find out what he or she is allergic to? Parents should be aware of some key signs.

If your child is continually ill with varying disorders, particularly middle ear infections, and if allergies run in your family, you should suspect allergies. Before taking action, however, it is essential to have the child checked by your family doctor to make sure there is no other condition that needs a different form of treatment. The doctor may refer you to an allergist if no other problems are found.

Children with a family history of allergies are a definite risk group because susceptibility to allergies has a strong genetic element. Boys develop allergies more often than girls do. This is particularly the case for attention deficit disorder, which some practitioners believe is a common symptom of hidden food allergy in children.

## KEY MARKERS FOR ALLERGY
Allergies may cause multiple symptoms that affect different systems of the body. The presence of multiple symptoms is one of the key indications that an allergy underlies a child's condition. If a child is affected by

## SYMPTOMS OF ALLERGY AND INTOLERANCE

There is an extensive range of symptoms that can be related to allergies and intolerances to foods or agents in the environment. Remember, though, that many of these symptoms may have causes other than allergy or intolerance.

| SYMPTOM GROUP | ACTUAL CONDITIONS |
|---|---|
| Gut problems | Diarrhea, constipation, recurrent stomach pains, colic in babies, feeding difficulties, itching anus, recurrent vomiting or feeling of sickness, mouth ulcers, poor appetite, food cravings |
| Brain/mood problems | Recurrent headaches, dizziness, poor concentration, hyperactivity, fidgeting, night waking, unexplained temper tantrums, attention deficit disorder, depression, seizures, restlessness, disturbed sleep, balance problems, persistent lethargy |
| Urinary/genital systems | Vaginal itching/discharge, sore genitals, frequent urinating, bed-wetting |
| Breathing problems | Blocked or runny nose, nosebleeds, pain in the front of the face (sinus pain), snoring, catarrh, middle ear infections, wheezing, asthma |
| Skin problems | Eczema, recurrent allergy rashes, itching skin, increased sweating |
| Joints and muscles | Recurrent joint pains, muscle aching, muscle weakness, cramps |
| General | Increased thirst, recurrent unexplained high temperatures, swollen lymph glands, nightmares, talking/walking in sleep, obesity, unexplained weight loss |

only one or two of these symptoms it is less likely that the problems are caused by an allergy, although some conditions, such as asthma, may occur in isolation.

Food allergies and intolerances have their own particular markers; excessive thirst is one indicator, being present in 95 percent of cases, and craving for a particular food is often a useful clue. Conversely, a strong aversion to the taste or smell of a particular food may indicate one to avoid.

## Diagnosis

The initial diagnosis of allergy as a cause of a child's symptoms is based on recognizing the symptom patterns described above. Then the same procedures—often laborious and inconvenient—must be applied as with adults (see Chapter 1). Laboratory tests, such as RAST, are useful for confirming some inhalant allergies but cannot help determine food allergies

For full and proper diagnosis, a detailed history is essential. This may be followed by taking precautions against house dust mites, molds, or animals, or instituting elimination diets and food challenges. These are the only truly reliable methods.

### TREATING A CHILD'S ALLERGY

Most of the principles of environmental management for adults also apply to allergic children. It is essential to consider all the places in which a child spends time, including home, school, a relative's or divorced parent's house, and the family car.

Avoiding allergens may require major changes in lifestyle and diet. The results can be enormously worthwhile, but for a child the restrictions can be distressing, damaging to social relations, and very difficult to put into practice. Sometimes such measures can be counterproductive because stressed and upset children are more prone to allergic attacks, particularly asthma. It is essential to help a child understand the need for adjustments and enlist the cooperation not only of the child but also relatives and friends.

## Planning major changes

When contemplating major changes in your environment, plan ahead. For instance, if you are moving to another house, check the area thoroughly from the point of view of an allergy sufferer and try to stay nearby for a trial period. If you are planning to get a pet, arrange for your child to visit the shop or owner daily for three weeks first, so you can check for an allergic reaction.

## Airborne allergens

House dust mites, molds, and dander from pets are the major airborne allergens, with pollen becoming more important as a child grows older. Chemical allergens, such as formaldehyde, are particularly implicated in asthma and allergic rhinitis. Even if your child's allergy is to a food rather than an airborne allergen, it is still important to reduce his or her exposure to airborne allergens because they increase the "allergen load," or total stress on an allergic child's already overstretched immune system.

### YOUR CHILD'S DIET

If it is established that your child has a food allergy or intolerance, then his or her diet will have to be modified. What degree of change do you need to implement? Is total avoidance always necessary?

Some young people are unable to tolerate even minute amounts of a trigger food and will have to avoid it completely. A case in point is a child who develops anaphylaxis after exposure to peanuts or even just a trace of them. Such a child needs careful monitoring by parents, relatives, teachers, and the parents of his or her friends. Many other youngsters have a degree of tolerance to a food and can eat small amounts occasionally without developing severe symptoms. Often a child starts off very sensitive and develops tolerance over time.

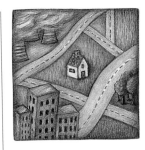

*TROUBLESOME NEIGHBORS*
*If you are serious about avoiding sources of trouble, check out a new area thoroughly before moving there. Avoid obvious problem spots, such as chemical plants or fields that are sprayed.*

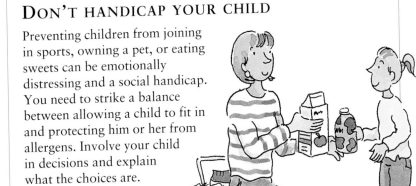

## DON'T HANDICAP YOUR CHILD

Preventing children from joining in sports, owning a pet, or eating sweets can be emotionally distressing and a social handicap. You need to strike a balance between allowing a child to fit in and protecting him or her from allergens. Involve your child in decisions and explain what the choices are.

*PROVIDE ALTERNATIVES*
*Instead of just saying no, suggest an alternative, such as juice instead of a milk shake.*

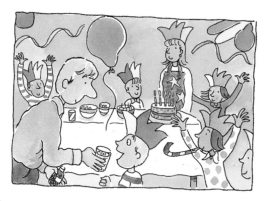

## Getting your child's help

Successfully modifying your child's diet depends on getting his or her full cooperation. This means that you must explain why the changes are being made. If anaphylaxis is not a risk, you might even allow a lapse in the diet, so that your child begins to recognize the association between what is eaten and the unpleasant consequences.

For children who can't avoid eating a forbidden food occasionally, a preventive oral preparation of cromolyn sodium, taken just prior to the lapse, may reduce the reaction.

## Balancing your child's diet

Simply excluding additives (see pages 94 and 96) from a child's diet can be done without any harm to nutrition, but more complex diets will require the advice of a dietitian or nutritionist to help ensure that the diet has no deficiencies in vitamins, minerals, or other nutrients.

### ANTIFUNGAL THERAPY

Antifungal therapy is a controversial approach to the management of allergies, but some specialists argue that it is a helpful alternative to keeping a child on a permanently restricted diet.

## What is it?

Antifungal therapy is based on the theory that yeast and fungal microorganisms in the gut cause symptoms of hidden food allergy and intolerance, either by acting as allergens themselves or by producing toxic fermentation products. The therapy is based on a diet involving the exclusion of sugars, yeast extracts, and fermented products.

In addition to these dietary controls, a naturopath might use herbal remedies like garlic, supplements of vitamins B and C, and live yogurt or other cultures of friendly bacteria (see page 89).

## Who can it help?

This therapy is most likely to be effective in children who have a history of frequent episodes of oral thrush (*Candida albicans* infection), who have had repeated antibiotic treatment, or whose parents are prone to candidiasis. It is important for the doctor or therapist to confirm that yeast, and not bacterial, overgrowth is responsible for the problems. This can be done with some simple laboratory tests.

## The role of antifungal drugs

Although a very strict diet is often recommended for adults, many children respond to a less strenuous dietary regimen combined with treatment with an antifungal drug. If the treatment is effective, it may have to be continued for several months.

A naturopath would favor a gentler antifungal preparation of caprylic acid, a fatty acid derived from coconut oil.

### WHAT THE CHILD CAN DO

Youngsters are often the best guardians of their own diets, once they are aware of what makes them feel unwell. Older children may be able to keep their own records of symptoms to help with identification of the triggers. Many young people are also good at avoiding environments that don't suit them; sometimes they are the strongest critics of their parents' smoking habits.

The most difficult children are those whose need for a special diet is not identified until they are 10 years old. By this age they are very resistant to change. Early identification of allergies and intolerances in a child is thus very important.

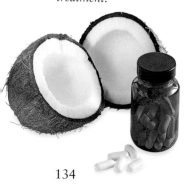

## Pathway to health

Excluding cow's milk from the diet is a common antiallergy measure, but it often causes parents anxiety over whether their child will suffer from a deficiency of calcium. Soy milk fortified with calcium or calcium supplements recommended by your doctor or a nutritionist can be acceptable substitutes, if they are tolerated. Always check with a doctor or dietitian before making major changes in your child's diet.

## Easing a Child's Asthma Attack with

# Relaxation

*The most effective way to help a child in the event of an asthma attack is to be prepared for one before it happens. Knowing what to do and when will reassure and calm both you and your child, which could be your most important contribution.*

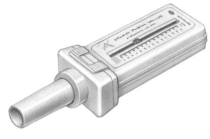

**PEAK FLOW METER**
*A peak flow meter is an easy-to-use tool for measuring the constriction of the bronchi. Changes can serve as an early warning of an attack or indicate how well medication is working.*

During an asthma attack the airways become constricted and fill with mucus (called bronchospasm), making it difficult for a child to breathe out, rather than in. Nonetheless, the worst thing any sufferer can do is panic, which may worsen the attack. It is important for you to stay calm and reassure the child; the presence of a relaxed, confident adult may be the most effective calming influence. You must also assess the severity of the attack; a severe one will require medical attention, so

before progressing further with self-help efforts, check for some warning signs. The most obvious one is cyanosis—a blue tinge to the lips and tongue. A peak flow meter can help in gauging severity. If you suspect the attack is severe, get medical help as soon as possible, either from a doctor or at the nearest emergency room or department. While waiting for help, get the child into the correct position (see below) and keep him or her calm. Clear the room and minimize distractions. Prevent fumes or smoke

from worsening the child's condition. Get the child to breathe slowly, concentrating on breathing out. After an acute attack, even one that was successfully controlled, you should have your child checked by a doctor to see if additional treatment is needed.

## POSITION YOUR CHILD CORRECTLY

During an asthma attack, get your child to sit down and lean forward, ideally with something to lean on. Don't make him or her lie down.

*LEAN FORWARD*
*A child uses the muscles around the chest to help with breathing during an asthma attack. Leaning forward helps them work better.*

Soothe the child with words of encouragement and remain as calm as possible.

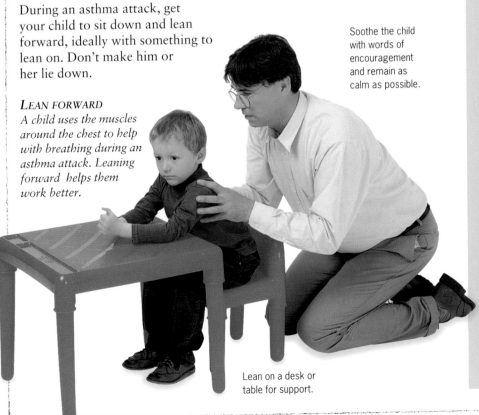

Lean on a desk or table for support.

### MEDICATION

Administering medication promptly and accurately is crucial in controlling an asthma attack. Familiarize yourself with your child's medications and make sure everyone in the household knows where they are kept and how they are used.

Attacks are treated with a bronchodilator administered with an inhaler or nebulizer. Two puffs should increase airflow within 15 minutes. If the child fails to respond, repeat the dose. If that has no effect, call 911 or take the child to a hospital. Emergency treatment there may include administration of oxygen and a corticosteroid or an intravenous injection of aminophylline (a bronchodilator in the xanthine group).

# HYPERACTIVITY AND FOOD ALLERGIES

*A disorder often linked with childhood allergy is hyperactivity, or attention deficit disorder. It can hinder a child's development, but may be helped by changes in diet.*

## SYMPTOMS OF ADHD

A child suffering from ADHD commonly exhibits many of these symptoms.

▶ *Is hyperactive and excitable; talks too fast and excessively.*

▶ *Constantly fidgets.*

▶ *Does not listen when spoken to.*

▶ *Has difficulty paying attention; is easily distracted.*

▶ *Is disruptive and difficult in school.*

▶ *Is impulsive. Has explosive mood changes.*

▶ *Is aggressive, quick to anger, and often depressed.*

▶ *Is clumsy and poorly coordinated.*

▶ *Has a poor self-image.*

▶ *Has disturbed sleep.*

Hyperactivity is just one aspect of a syndrome known variously as attention deficit hyperactivity disorder (ADHD), attention deficit spectrum, hyperkinesis, or minimal brain dysfunction. All describe essentially the same behavioral disorder that has a range of related symptoms and only minor differences.

### HOW IS THE SYNDROME DIAGNOSED?

Media interest in ADHD has given the impression that it is a well-defined condition for which there is a single diagnosis. This is not the case. Many people prefer to use the term "attention deficit spectrum" to reflect that the disorder can vary in severity and range of symptoms. The grouping of symptoms associated with ADHD can be attributed to at least 14 possible diagnoses, each needing a different approach. High among these possibilities are food intolerance, food allergy (in particular to additives), or a nutritional deficiency. Although powerful drugs are available for controlling the disorder and are widely used in North America, it makes sense to exclude the allergy possibilities before risking side effects from a drug therapy that does not address the root causes of the problem.

Children who are likely to benefit from dietary treatment can usually be identified using the same criteria as those for any food allergy or intolerance—by observing the symptoms, the timing and combination of symptoms, and the response of the affected child to an elimination diet.

### WHAT PROOF IS THERE THAT ALLERGIES ARE INVOLVED?

The role played by food sensitivity in the behavioral problems of hyperactive children is an ongoing controversial topic. There are still many skeptics, despite some excellent studies that have established the benefits that dietary treatment can produce in some youngsters with ADHD. One of them, conducted at the Great Ormond Street Children's Hospital in London, found that severely hyperactive children showed marked improvement after the introduction of a "few foods" diet—a regimen stricter than the Stone Age diet (see pages 84–85), excluding most common allergenic foods. Some of the children were given double-blind food challenges to see whether any particular food trigger could be identified. A statistically significant number were shown to have increased symptoms after such challenges, thus proving the involvement of food.

There is continuing debate over how many hyperactive children can be helped through diet, although a 1994 American study in the *Annals of Allergy* suggested that 74 percent of children with ADHD referred to a clinic could be helped by dietary changes.

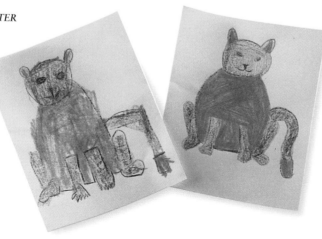

***BEFORE AND AFTER*** *One sign of improvement in hyperactive children is better drawing skills, reflecting improved concentration and dexterity.*

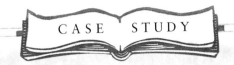

# A Hyperactive Child

*Hyperactivity is just one aspect of a debilitating condition known by various names, including attention deficit spectrum and attention deficit hyperactivity disorder (ADHD). Children suffering from this disorder generally exhibit high levels of nervous activity, have difficulty at school, readily get into fights, and find it impossible to sit still.*

John is five years old and has a history of chronic medical complaints. He has had a constant runny nose and frequent ear infections for at least two years, and does not sleep well. His teachers at school have complained of his frequent misbehavior in class and his poor ability to pay attention and to participate in quiet activities.

John's mother took him to see the family doctor, who noticed that he looked pale and had dark rings under his eyes but that he was full of energy and constantly on the go—climbing onto chairs, picking things up and dropping them—and was easily distracted. The doctor also noted that John's coordination was not what it should be for a child of his age.

## WHAT SHOULD JOHN'S MOTHER DO?

The doctor tentatively diagnosed ADHD but recommended a CT scan and an electroencephalogram to rule out structural brain damage. He also had John seen by a child psychologist. The examinations confirmed the family doctor's initial diagnosis, and he advised treatment with the drug Ritalin. However, John's mother had read about food allergies and wanted to try an elimination diet first. She consulted with an allergist, who advised first cutting out foods high in additives and sugar, then milk, wheat, and eggs. If his symptoms improved, they would then try some food challenges to identify which foods were responsible for the condition.

### HEALTH
*Food allergies can cause various chronic conditions, including frequent infections of the middle ear in children. These can act as markers for allergic disorders.*

### DIET
*Milk, wheat, and eggs are common allergy triggers. Additives such as flavorings or colorings, along with high levels of refined sugar, are particularly implicated in ADHD.*

### CHILDREN
*Disruptive behavior along with other symptoms may indicate a food allergy or intolerance.*

## Action Plan

### DIET
*Adopt a special diet: eliminate soft drinks, sweetened juices, sweets, and processed foods with additives. One by one cut out foods containing milk, wheat, and eggs.*

### CHILDREN
*Tell teachers, grandparents, and the parents of the child's friends about the special diet, and make sure they know how important it is to stick to it.*

### HEALTH
*Keep a diary of symptoms, situations, and foods to identify triggers that should be avoided.*

## HOW THINGS TURNED OUT FOR JOHN

After three months on an elimination diet, John's nose stopped running. Food challenges showed he was allergic to wheat and a few food additives. His sleep improved, as did his behavior at home and school, and he was able to concentrate better and interact more appropriately with other children. His teachers were pleased with his new attentiveness and reported that his speech and drawing skills were improving rapidly.

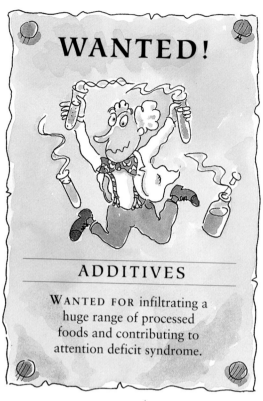

# WANTED!

## ADDITIVES

**WANTED FOR** infiltrating a huge range of processed foods and contributing to attention deficit syndrome.

## PSYCHOLOGICAL FACTORS

In many cases where children demonstrate hyperactivity, impaired concentration, learning deficits, and difficult behavior, there is also evidence of a poor parent-child relationship. But parenting problems may be a result rather than a cause of difficulties: many children with a hidden food allergy or intolerance have been difficult from early infancy, presenting their parents with a child who cries a lot, disturbs their sleep perpetually, and does not often reciprocate their affection. Inevitably this beharior will affect the parents and siblings as well, impairing the process of attachment that is essential to good family relationships. This is why it is important to recognize when a child is suffering from ADHD at the earliest possible stage, before any lasting damage occurs. Then it is necessary to accept hyperactivity as a chronic condition that needs special attention.

## DEALING WITH HYPERACTIVITY

ADHD may have caused distress within the family, educational underachievement, and low self-esteem in the child prior to diagnosis. Thus, the problems created by ADHD may continue to cause emotional difficulties even after successful treatment. Professionals call these secondary emotional difficulties, and they can produce more stress and emotional disturbance, making the child even more vulnerable to allergy.

### Getting support

Parents and schools must work together to help a child adapt to dietary restrictions, and this may be hindered if teachers or relatives are skeptical. Parent support groups can be very helpful for obtaining practical advice and information.

### Managing the problem

There are many things parents can do to help a child overcome hyperactivity. Especially important is maintaining an orderly, calm home environment. Keep a consistent daily routine with specific times for meals, naps, play, snacks, and going to bed. Limit television viewing and permit child-suitable, nonviolent programs only. Allocate an open space for active play, but also encourage quiet activities with age-appropriate picture books, games, and puzzles. Always give praise for obeying or playing quietly.

# ADHD AND FAMILY DYNAMICS

The symptoms of ADHD interact with psychological and emotional factors within the family. If left untreated these problems can feed back on one another, causing a negative spiral of worsening behavioral and emotional difficulties.

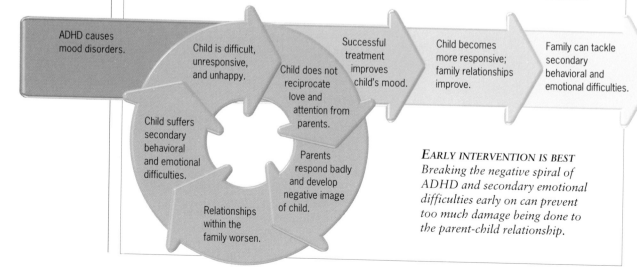

ADHD causes mood disorders.

Child is difficult, unresponsive, and unhappy.

Child does not reciprocate love and attention from parents.

Successful treatment improves child's mood.

Child becomes more responsive; family relationships improve.

Family can tackle secondary behavioral and emotional difficulties.

Child suffers secondary behavioral and emotional difficulties.

Parents respond badly and develop negative image of child.

Relationships within the family worsen.

***EARLY INTERVENTION IS BEST***
*Breaking the negative spiral of ADHD and secondary emotional difficulties early on can prevent too much damage being done to the parent-child relationship.*

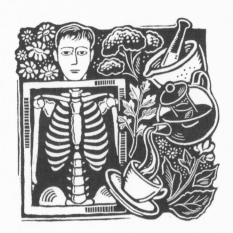

# CHAPTER 9

# A DIRECTORY OF ALLERGIC DISORDERS

*Allergic reactions have been implicated as the hidden cause of a host of conditions, many of which are chronic and incapacitating. Avoidance measures and elimination diets can often help, when doctors have excluded other causes and are at a loss as to how to proceed.*

# ALLERGY OR ILLNESS?

*Allergies are responsible for a wide range of symptoms, but most of these can have other causes as well. How can you tell if your symptoms are part of an allergic condition?*

## COULD YOU BE SUFFERING FROM AN ALLERGY?

If your doctor cannot help you, ask yourself some basic questions:

▶ *Are your symptoms chronic or persistent? Do you have many unrelated symptoms? These are classic markers of Type B allergies.*

▶ *Do you recall a time when you were free of symptoms? If your symptoms cleared up while you were away or on a different diet, it could be a useful clue about possible triggers.*

▶ *Have you noticed any regular correlations between your symptoms and certain situations or times? For instance, if they are worse in the morning, it could be that high levels of dust mite allergen or chemicals in your bedroom are to blame.*

Is it an allergy or illness? This simple question goes to the heart of many controversies about allergy. The conventional medical view restricts the disorders caused by allergy to those in which the immune system is clearly involved. These conditions can usually be confirmed with well-established diagnostic tests. It is possible, however, that many other chronic illnesses are due to allergy, although the links are harder to detect.

### CHRONIC ILLNESS CAUSED BY ALLERGY

Chronic illnesses caused by allergy have three main features. First, the relationship between allergen and illness is often hidden. Second, patients are often affected by more than one substance and may react only when triggers are encountered in combination. Third, patients experience multiple symptoms. If you have migraine and irritable bowel syndrome, for instance, or rhinitis along with mood changes, you are likely to have an allergy. Also, if your symptoms are repeatedly worse during a certain part of the menstrual cycle or when you are under stress, allergies may be involved.

The hidden nature of this sort of allergic reaction can prevent sufferers from realizing what is happening and so they continue to expose themselves to the triggers, leading to the development of chronic, often multiple symptoms. Some people may be given a

*DOCTOR KNOWS BEST*
*You should check with your doctor if you have been feeling repeatedly ill. If he or she cannot identify the cause it might be worth considering allergies.*

standard medical diagnosis, often more than one, but there may not be any abnormal physical findings or laboratory results.

Patients who have chronic allergies may also suffer multiple adverse drug reactions because they are prone to developing side effects with drug treatments, particularly when several different drugs are prescribed.

### WHAT SHOULD YOU DO IF YOU SUSPECT ALLERGIES?

People who suspect that allergies are causing their symptoms should consult their family physician before taking steps themselves to find out what is wrong, because overlooking other diagnoses could be dangerous, delaying appropriate treatment. After ruling out serious diseases that could

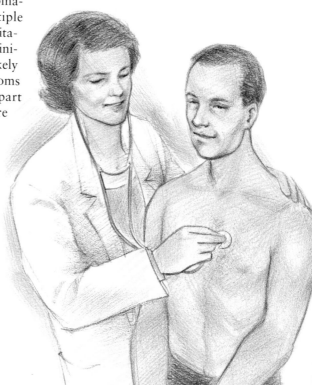

## FACTORS THAT INDICATE ALLERGY

Allergy is more likely to be the cause of your symptoms if you react to medicines or there is a history of allergy in your family. Allergy is also suggested by a number of features that are characteristic of allergic conditions and help to distinguish them from other illnesses. These features may be given a conventional interpretation, but can be indicative of allergies nonetheless.

| IF YOUR SYMPTOMS... | EVEN IF... |
|---|---|
| ... are variable | ... you have not noticed a clear link between symptoms and changes in activity, place, or time. |
| ... are multiple | ... a standard diagnosis has been given for each. |
| ... respond to steroids | ... your symptoms have been treated with antibiotics or other drugs. |
| ... differ in severity with activity, place, or time | ... they are also stress related or get worse premenstrually. |

be responsible for the symptoms, investigations can be started to look for triggers that might be provoking an allergic reaction.

### THE PROBLEM OF MULTIPLE SYMPTOMS

Patients with Type B allergies usually complain of multiple symptoms. Detailed medical histories, which look at how often a patient with a Type B allergy has each symptom, show that most of them have 5 to 10 symptoms, and 20 to 30 symptoms are not uncommon. Many are nonspecific, for instance fatigue, sweating, insomnia, fluid retention, muscle pain, and weight fluctuation. Others are typical of eczema, asthma, rhinitis, migraine, and irritable bowel syndrome, or even of such conditions as arthritis or old injuries. When consulting their doctors, such patients are usually conscious of time constraints and they may concentrate on the major symptoms, leaving out minor ones entirely; this omission can lead to a misdiagnosis.

Patients with long-term multiple symptoms for which no disease or other physical cause can be determined are often diagnosed with somatization syndrome, a condition in which physical symptoms result from psychological pain. In some of these cases it could be allergies that are causing persistent Type B symptoms.

### PROOF FOR THE ROLE OF ALLERGIES

The medical histories of thousands of people strongly suggest that many symptoms suffered by polysymptomatic patients are provoked by environmental factors, and that when these factors are removed or controlled, the majority of the symptoms are relieved, either wholly or in part.

Those opposed to the allergy hypothesis argue that patients get better because of the extra attention they receive with this sort of therapy, or that the treatments simply have a placebo effect—patients believe that the treatment will work, and the psychological boost helps to counteract the psychological causes of the illness.

At the moment the anecdotal evidence can be interpreted either way, but there is a growing body of evidence from properly controlled studies that supports the theories of the environmentalists. If they are right, then there is little doubt that allergies and related problems like intolerances could be responsible for a wide range of illnesses.

### HOW TO USE THIS SECTION

The directory of disorders on the following pages covers the most common health problems that can be linked with sensitivities or allergies, particularly to foods. The conditions are grouped according to the body systems that they affect.

▶ *Skin and joint disorders: skin inflammation, acne, soreness of the mouth and lips, arthritis.*

▶ *Gastrointestinal disorders: celiac disease, colic, constipation, diarrhea, irritable bowel syndrome, obesity.*

▶ *Nervous disorders: insomnia, anxiety, mood disturbances, fatigue, migraine and other headaches.*

▶ *Genitourinary disorders: kidney and bladder problems, infertility, vaginal inflammation.*

▶ *Respiratory disorders: sinusitis, ear problems, hay fever, asthma.*

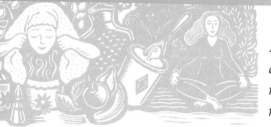

# Skin and Joint Disorders

*An environmental approach to treating skin and joint disorders can help clear up chronic problems that may not respond to conventional medical treatment. Using natural remedies to soothe symptoms can reduce reliance on drugs.*

## SKIN INFLAMMATION

Hives (urticaria or nettle rash), eczema, and dermatitis are types of skin inflammation that can be caused by allergies. Hives are a form of intensely itchy rash, made up of multiple wheals that usually have a red edge and a white center and last from a few hours to a day, but they may keep appearing in crops.

Eczema and dermatitis, terms that are often used interchangeably, are characterized by dryness, flaking, and cracking of the skin, accompanied by itching. Sometimes small bubbles form under the skin and these may break open and weep.

**Causes** Hives can be provoked by physical factors such as exercise or excessive cold or heat, but like eczema and dermatitis they often represent an allergic reaction, either from direct contact with an allergen or through eating or inhaling one.

**Treatment** Hives are usually managed with antihistamines, but corticosteroids are sometimes prescribed. Standard medical treatment for eczema involves the use of moisturizing agents and corticosteroids, usually applied as a cream or lotion but sometimes taken orally. In patients who react to an ingredient in skin cream—lanolin or a preservative, for instance—even a corticosteroid cream can exacerbate

eczema. Scratching also worsens the condition. Putting mittens on young children will limit the amount of damage they can do with scratching.

Supplements of zinc or evening primrose oil often help. The oil can be swallowed or rubbed on the skin. Other remedies include calendula cream for dryness, chickweed ointment for itchiness, and chamomile cream for both. Chinese medicine and homeopathy both have good track records in treating allergic skin problems, particularly eczema.

Neither conventional nor alternative treatments of symptoms get to the root of the problem, however; the best strategy is to avoid the triggers.

### PREVENTION

▶ In some forms of eczema, reducing exposure to house dust mites, molds, and animal allergens may result in marked improvement. Everything the patient comes into contact with must be considered, including laundry detergents, fabrics, nickel in jewelry, and additives in drugs.

▶ Hidden food allergies should be considered if avoiding inhaled and contact allergens does not work. In children with severe eczema, food challenges should be used only under medical supervision because serious reactions can occur.

### MAKING A SOOTHING CHAMOMILE CREAM

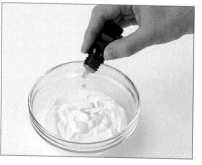

**1** *Mix 100 ml (3½ oz) of hypo-allergenic cream with 4 to 6 drops of essential oil of chamomile. Blend them thoroughly.*

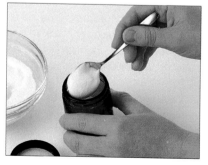

**2** *Spoon the mixture into a sterilized dark glass jar, to protect the contents from the light, and seal and label it with the date and contents.*

# ACNE

Acne is a skin disorder manifested by whiteheads, blackheads, pimples, and cysts, mainly on the face, chest, and back. These result from a buildup of sebum mixed with dead skin cells, bacteria, and other debris that clogs pores and leads to inflammation of the hair follicles and sebaceous glands.

**Causes** Some medications can cause acne, and it can be made worse by oil-based cosmetics that block the ducts. Foods do not trigger acne but certain ones can make it worse.

**Treatment** Acne is often treated with benzoyl peroxide, which is antibacterial and exfoliating. (Tea tree oil is said to yield the same results without the side effects.) Topical or oral antibiotics may be prescribed for persistent acne and retinoid drugs for severe cases. A daily dietary approach includes drinking at least eight glasses of water, eating five to eight servings of vegetables and fruits plus whole-grain breads and cereals, and avoiding foods containing sugar and iodine.

*SPOT TREATMENT*
*Herbalists may advise infusions (teas) of dandelion, nettle, or burdock for acne treatment. These herbs are thought to remove toxins and cleanse the blood.*

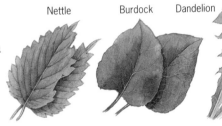

Nettle          Burdock          Dandelion

### PREVENTION

▶ Do not put oil on your face, including oil-based cosmetics and lotions.

▶ If you suspect certain medications or foods may be contributing to your acne, stop using the drugs and try an elimination diet.

▶ Naturopaths recommend reducing intake of dairy products, nuts, citrus fruits, sugar, white bread, red meat, caffeine, and alcohol. Useful dietary supplements include zinc, taken at night apart from other nutrients, and vitamins A, B, and C. (Pregnant women or those planning a pregnancy should not take more than 1,200 mcg, or 4,000 IU of vitamin A a day.)

# SORE MOUTH AND LIPS

Soreness around the mouth and lips can be caused by mouth ulcers, cold sores, or cracks at the corners of the mouth (angular stomatitis). In some patients who complain of sore or burning mouth or lips, however, there is nothing abnormal to be seen, even when the symptoms are so bad that these people cannot tolerate eating anything hot or spicy.

Marked swelling of the mouth and lips can be a sign of angioedema. If it involves the tongue or throat, it could be dangerous; medical attention should be sought immediately.

**Causes** Mouth ulcers can be caused by deficiencies of iron or the B vitamins in the diet, problems with dentures, or a reaction to an ingredient in toothpaste or a mouthwash. In rare cases they can result from allergic reactions to fillings. Where there is no obvious cause, hidden food allergies are often to blame. Cold sores are caused by the herpes simplex virus, but the virus may be dormant until triggered by ill health, stress, or allergic illness. Pain with no visible outbreak may be an allergic reaction to food.

**Treatment** Medication can be given to alleviate symptoms but may not be much help. Antiviral creams such as acyclovir can prevent cold sores if used as soon as the warning tingle of an imminent attack is noticed. Herbal remedies may help relieve mouth ulcers. You can make a soothing mouthwash by mixing a couple of drops each of geranium and lavender oil in a tumbler of water. A cooled infusion of licorice combined with extract of sage makes a mildly antiseptic mouthwash.

### PREVENTION

▶ Ulcers, sores, and conditions in which there is discomfort with no apparent physical outbreak will often respond to an elimination diet or avoidance of common chemical triggers, some of which are often found in commercial toothpastes and mouthwashes.

▶ Naturopaths suggest avoiding foods rich in arginine—such as nuts, chocolate, peas, cereals, and garlic—and increasing intake of fish, cheese, brewer's yeast, and yogurt. Recovery can be quick if all triggers are avoided, but may take up to four weeks.

*LIP SERVICE*
*Geranium oil, diluted with sweet almond oil, can be rubbed in as an aromatherapy treatment for sore mouth and lips.*

## ARTHRITIS

Arthritis is an inflammatory condition that can affect any joint in the body, including those in the spine. It usually starts in the lining of the joint, the synovial membrane, but may spread to cartilage and bone. It causes symptoms of pain, swelling, stiffness, and limited movement. In severe cases, it leads to long-term joint damage and deformity.

**Causes** There are numerous types of arthritis; some result from infections, others are due to metabolic disorders, and many are of unknown origin. The two most common types are rheumatoid arthritis and osteoarthritis. Normal wear and tear is thought to be the major cause of osteoarthritis. Rheumatoid arthritis is an autoimmune response. Some allergists believe that allergic reactions—in particular hidden food allergies—may be involved in rheumatoid arthritis, as well as some other types of arthritis, a view that is gaining acceptance because studies

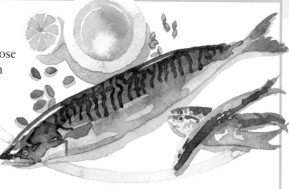

*ESSENTIAL FATTY ACIDS*
*You can get essential fatty acids from a variety of sources, including evening primrose oil supplements, oily fish, such as mackerel or sardines, pumpkin seeds, or oil from flaxseed, also called linseed.*

increasingly show that changing eating habits can reduce the severity of the disease in some people.

**Treatment** Conventional therapy includes nonsteroidal anti-inflammatory medications and corticosteroids. However, these drugs treat only symptoms, not root causes, and corticosteroids suppress the immune system, which can cause side effects.

### PREVENTION

▶ In many cases of arthritis hidden food allergy plays a part in provoking the inflammatory process. Identifying the trigger foods with an elimination diet can be beneficial, although the benefits will vary among individuals. The foods that commonly exacerbate arthritis are dairy products, grains, coffee, nuts, and foods in the nightside family—including potatoes, tomatoes, eggplants, and sweet peppers—but any food can potentially cause problems.

▶ Food additives, chemical pollutants, and inhaled allergens can also be responsible.

▶ A sufficient amount of essential fatty acids in the diet is also important. Evening primrose oil (see page 108) contains the essential fatty acid gamma-linolenic acid (GLA), which is an essential precursor of prostaglandin E— an important anti-inflammatory substance that helps to limit allergic reactions. GLA is also found in borage oil. Other types of essential fatty acid are found in oily fish, such as mackerel, flaxseed (linseed ) oil, and pumpkin seeds. Try to increase the amounts of these foods in your diet.

▶ It may be worthwhile taking a general vitamin and mineral supplement as well, especially if you are on a restricted diet.

▶ Being overweight is a major risk factor for arthritis, and losing excess weight can be of significant benefit to sufferers. Elimination diets to exclude allergenic foods can help in two ways. First, they tend to be healthful diets, with more attention paid to keeping nutrients balanced. Second, being overweight is common in allergic individuals and may resolve itself if the triggers are found and avoided.

---

## ARTHRITIS AND JOINTS

In any joint, like the hip joint shown below, two bones articulate against each other. To keep the joint lubricated and cushioned, it is sealed in a capsule lined with synovial membrane and filled with synovial fluid. The articulating surfaces of the bone are covered in smooth, protective, friction-reducing cartilage.

*RHEUMATOID ARTHRITIS*
*In rheumatoid arthritis, the synovial membrane becomes inflamed and thickened, and the inflammation often spreads to the cartilage and bone. The movement of the joint is thus impeded, and it may become twisted and misshapen.*

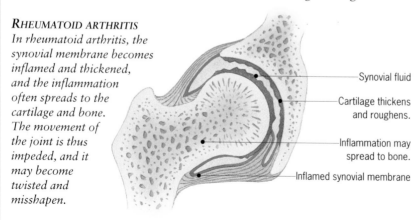

Synovial fluid

Cartilage thickens and roughens.

Inflammation may spread to bone.

Inflamed synovial membrane

# Gastrointestinal Disorders

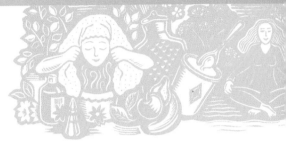

*Although food allergies and intolerances can cause problems for almost every system of the body, they are particularly associated with digestive and gut disorders. These create discomfort and pain and can affect nutrient absorption and general health.*

## CELIAC DISEASE

Celiac disease is a chronic condition involving the small bowel (the upper intestine). It is characterized by poor absorption of nutrients, diarrhea, weight loss, mouth ulcers, and sometimes a characteristic skin lesion called dermatitis herpetiformis.

**Causes** This condition is caused by sensitivity to gluten, which is contained in wheat, barley, rye, and in smaller quantities in some other grains. Even small doses of gluten can damage the intestinal walls in celiac sufferers. Celiac disease usually starts in childhood but can occur at any age. Though not precisely an allergy, celiac results from an immunological reaction— a protein in gluten combines with antibodies in the digestive tract.

**Treatment** No medication will make any specific improvement in celiac disease. Strict avoidance of gluten normally brings complete relief from symptoms; most sufferers can use rice, corn, buckwheat, and sometimes oats as substitutes for the restricted grains. A registered dietitian can help plan a suitable diet and may also recommend a vitamin and mineral supplement to counter any nutritional deficiencies. Herbs such as peppermint and ginger aid digestive function and soothe the sensitive intestinal walls.

## COLIC

Colic is a condition in which a healthy infant regularly cries for prolonged periods; the problem most often begins a few days after birth and ends by three months of age. The cause is usually unknown, but milk allergy should be investigated, especially if crying is accompanied by diarrhea or excessive gassiness.

**Causes** If milk allergy is the cause, it most often occurs in a bottle-fed infant but can also strike a breast-fed baby when the mother passes on allergens in foods she has eaten.

*DILL SEEDS*
*Dill seeds can be used to make a soothing infusion for colicky babies.*

**Treatment** Feeding your baby a spoonful of fennel, chamomile, or dill infusion may help to relieve pain caused by gas. To make an infusion, pour 1 cup boiling water over 1 teaspoon dried leaves or ½ teaspoon crushed dill or fennel seed, leave for 5 minutes, strain, and allow to cool.

## CONSTIPATION

Frequency of bowel movement varies among individuals, but anyone who has hard, dry stools or difficulty in passing stools in addition to infrequent ones is clearly constipated.

**Causes**  The major reasons for constipation are too little exercise and eating too little fiber, but other causes can range from depression, to irritable bowel syndrome, to cancer. Constipation can also result from allergies, especially if it alternates with periods of diarrhea and occurs along with other symptoms, such as abdominal bloating or gas.

**Treatment**  A high-fiber diet, an increase in exercise, and a fluid intake of at least eight glasses a day, if possible, are the most effective steps. However, some people report that their symptoms become worse if they eat bran, which suggests a possible wheat allergy. Avoiding wheat products and eating different cereals may be effective. If there is no improvement, a doctor should be consulted to exclude serious organic causes, such as cancer. Over-the-counter laxatives should be limited to short-term use only, and the same applies to laxative herbal remedies like infusions of fenugreek, flaxseed (linseed), or vervain.

*STOMACH MASSAGE*
*Massaging your lower abdomen may help to relieve the symptoms of constipation. Rhythmically stroke the abdomen, using undulating pressure in a clockwise pattern around the navel.*

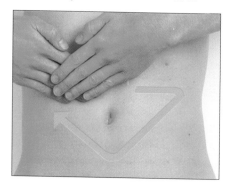

### PREVENTION

▶ A well-balanced diet high in fruits, vegetables, and whole grains is the most important approach to preventing constipation. However, a significant number of people with constipation have evidence of food intolerance and do not improve until the food or foods concerned are detected and avoided. Such individuals are commonly sensitive to several foods.

▶ In children, milk products are the most common triggers, whereas cereals are the major contributing factor in adults.

▶ A wide range of other foods may provoke constipation—even fruit, which is often eaten to increase the fiber content of the diet. If fruit makes the condition worse, avoid it and try drinking more water, eating fibrous foods that you can tolerate, and perhaps using supplements to compensate for missing nutrients.

## DIARRHEA

Diarrhea is a common condition, usually associated with 3 or more loose, runny movements a day, but in extreme cases up to 30 a day. The movements may contain undigested food, mucus, or blood.

**Causes**  There are many causes of diarrhea, the most common being infections and irritable bowel syndrome (see opposite page). Other factors include stress and enzyme deficiencies such as lactose intolerance. If diarrhea persists, serious causes must be considered, especially chronic inflammatory problems like Crohn's disease and ulcerative colitis. Diarrhea is also a common symptom of hidden food allergy, which may even play a role in these other diseases.

**Treatment**  Drugs like loperamide can be used to control diarrhea in the short term. Severe diarrhea, which upsets the balance of salts (electrolytes) in the blood, should be countered with rehydration salts, available from pharmacies, or a sports drink like Gatorade. Aromatherapy with lavender, chamomile, juniper, or sandalwood essential oils can help relieve stress; add 6 to 8 drops of one of these to your bath or put 2 or 3 drops in a bowl of steaming water, drape a towel over your head, and inhale the vapors. Other relaxing therapies, such as deep breathing, may bring relief in a case of stress-induced diarrea. A homeopath may recommend *Arsenicum*.

### PREVENTION

▶ Elimination diets to identify triggers and subsequent avoidance of the foods causing the problems are the most effective prevention for cases in which diarrhea is caused by hidden food allergy or irritable bowel syndrome. When other conditions are responsible, dietary measures may not be sufficient, and other medical intervention may be needed.

*TASTY TREATMENT*
*Taking a teaspoon of honey with one drop each of peppermint oil and white oak bark extract, every two hours, may help control diarrhea.*

# IRRITABLE BOWEL SYNDROME

Irritable bowel syndrome (IBS) is very common, especially in women; some researchers estimate that at least half of women of reproductive age may have IBS. The diagnosis is usually made after other diseases with similar symptoms have been ruled out. Typical symptoms are recurrent abdominal pain, bloating, gas, nausea, and constipation or diarrhea, sometimes alternating bouts of both. Some people also experience fatigue, headaches, and depression. In women symptoms are frequently worse just before menstruation.

**Causes** Although no specific cause has been found for IBS, it may be aggravated by food allergies or intolerances. An imbalance in the gut microorganisms, usually an overgrowth of fungi, may also be implicated. Such a condition is exacerbated by eating a lot of refined carbohydrates (sugars and white flours) and is more likely to occur

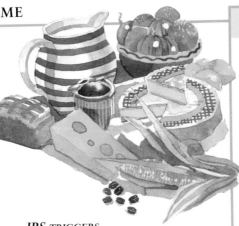

**IBS** TRIGGERS
*The main culprits tend to be wheat or corn, milk products, tea, coffee, onions, potatoes, and citrus fruit.*

after gut infections and the use of antibiotics. Stress is another factor that worsens IBS.

**Treatment** A doctor may prescribe drugs to quell abnormal muscle contractions and alleviate diarrhea. However, dietary measures and stress reduction are the mainstays of treatment. IBS responds well to

the detection and avoidance of foods that trigger symptoms. Identifying foods that help calm the condition can also be helpful. If constipation is a problem, adding more high-fiber foods, such as fruits, vegetables, nuts, seeds, and whole-grain cereals , to the diet should bring improvement. Anti-yeast treatment may be necessary for fungal overgrowth.

# OBESITY

Obesity is a major problem in North America, where calorie consumption is high and exercise is decreasing. A recent survey shows that 54 percent of Americans are overweight—about 97 million people—and 23 percent are obese. In Canada 40 percent of adults are overweight and, of these, some 28 percent are obese.

**Causes** Obesity has many causes, just one of which may be hidden food allergies, often indicated by fluid retention and cravings. Also, the most common allergenic foods—

wheat, eggs, and milk—are often ingredients of high-calorie foods.

**Treatment** To control obesity it is necessary to reduce calorie intake and increase activity levels at the same time. If these measures do not succeed, an elimination diet should be considered (see page 43), particularly if there are other symptoms. Weigh yourself in the morning and at night during the challenge period and avoid foods that cause a weight gain of more than 1 kilogram (2.2 pounds) over a day.

(see page 43)

CHAIN OF FOOD
*Allergies can act to increase weight in several ways, and these mechanisms may interact to exacerbate the problems.*

| Hidden food allergy causes cravings for allergenic food. | Cravings cause bingeing on high-calorie food triggers. | Fluid retention results, and general health deteriorates. | Sufferer is unwell and does less exercise; metabolic rate falls, reducing number of calories burned. |

# Nervous Disorders

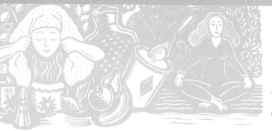

*The role of allergies in psychological disturbances and problems involving the central nervous system is controversial and the subject of much debate, but dietary and environmental measures are known to be effective in relieving some nervous disorders.*

## INSOMNIA

Insomnia is a catch-all term. It covers a variety of sleep-related problems, including difficulty in getting to sleep, awaking early, experiencing disturbed sleep (waking frequently during the night), and not feeling rested in the morning.

**Causes** Anything that induces stress, tension, anxiety, or physical discomfort can lead to insomnia. Too much caffeine is also a common factor, as are eating and drinking late at night.

Environmental causes are not unusual. Hidden food allergies especially sensitivities to food additives and contaminants, are known to produce insomnia. Exposure to volatile chemicals, particularly those from furniture and building materials (see Chapter 3) may also be to blame. House dust mite allergens, which are usually at their highest concentration in the bedroom, can be a causative agent as well. Pollens and molds are less likely to be responsible directly, but they may have an indirect effect by causing nasal obstruction, coughing, or wheezing.

**Treatment** A standard treatment for insomnia is a healthy diet of fresh foods, avoidance of those containing additives or a lot of sugar, and cutting back on drinks that contain caffeine. Other approaches include eating meals at regular times (not after seven at night), exercising regularly, and practicing relaxation techniques. Sedatives should not be used for more than a few days at a time.

There are many complementary remedies for insomnia. They include a few drops of lavender oil on your pillow at night, rosemary oil baths, mustard foot baths, and several traditional Chinese medicines. Homeopaths recommend *Coffea* to counteract mental restlessness.

A naturopathic treatment for insomnia is to wash your legs and feet in cold water before going to bed, followed by a relaxation routine. A simple technique you can practice in bed is progressive muscle relaxation. Get settled comfortably and start breathing deeply and steadily. Beginning at your toes, focus on a group of muscles, tense them, and then relax them, concentrating on the feelings this causes. From the feet, work up through your legs, arms, abdomen, chest, back, neck, and face.

*COOL AND RELAXING*
*Bathe your feet and legs in cold water for two to three minutes, then dry them carefully and lie on your bed.*

# ANXIETY

Anxiety is a normal emotional response to stress, but it may also occur when there is no reason to be anxious. It is often accompanied by symptoms like shortness of breath, hyperventilation, a feeling of panic, dizziness, and sweating.

**Causes** Anxiety attacks are associated with some psychological conditions, premenstrual tension, and thyroid problems. The attacks sometimes occur also in people who consume an excessive amount of caffeinated beverages.

Food intolerance and allergy may be involved in anxiety attacks that have no other obvious cause, and the attacks may coincide with the onset of menstruation or periods of stress. Patients who suffer from multiple chemical sensitivities can have anxiety attacks as a result of exposure to chemicals.

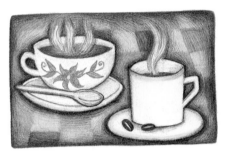

*CUT DOWN ON YOUR CAFFEINE*
*Caffeine intake should be reduced to a daily maximum of 50 mg—about one cup of tea or half a cup of coffee.*

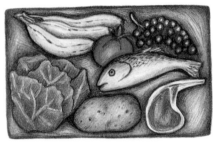

*BOOST YOUR FRESH FOODS*
*Eating more fruits, vegetables, fish, and meat will provide beneficial B vitamins, magnesium, and other minerals.*

## PREVENTION

▶ If an environmental cause is established, avoidance may prevent symptoms.

▶ Some patients find that they benefit from a vitamin and mineral supplement that includes the B vitamins, magnesium, and calcium.

▶ Training in breathing techniques can reduce susceptibility to asthma attacks and hyperventilation.

**Treatment** Counseling, reducing stress, and a controlled use of tranquilizers and antidepressants are the usual ways of dealing with the symptoms. Naturopaths advocate nutritional therapy, including the vitamin B complex and magnesium.

Try to reduce your exposure to chemicals and identify any food allergies using an elimination diet. Be prepared for panic attacks when doing food challenges and make sure you have help and support on hand.

# MOOD DISTURBANCES

Depression, aggression, anxiety, irritability, and hyperactivity in children have all been linked with allergies. Some researchers believe that allergic reactions may even be a factor in criminal behavior.

**Causes** Frequent mood changes are often attributed to genetic makeup, psychological problems, or stress, but allergic reactions to environmental factors and foods are often a cause. Foods and food additives are sometimes responsible for hyperactivity in children and irritability in adults. In young children milk, wheat, and citrus fruits are leading culprits. In older children food colorings and other additives are the most common causes but sugars, milk products, and other foods may also be responsible. In adults reactions to alcohol, cigarette smoke, coffee, and carbonated drinks containing additives are common causes of irritability. Some cases of depression have been shown to result from sensitivity to wheat and dairy products, but allergy to any food can be responsible. Deficiencies of the B vitamins may cause mental problems, including depression. Chemical fumes, including air fresheners, are also common culprits.

**Treatment** Although there are many drugs for their treatment, mood disturbances can be very difficult to control satisfactorily. Disturbances are often transient, lasting only a few hours, making control with medications difficult without producing unacceptable side effects. Drugs are widely used to treat hyperactive children with variable success and uncertain side effects. It is better to identify the triggers and avoid exposure if possible. Supplements of B vitamins and the minerals calcium, magnesium, and zinc can be helpful.

## PREVENTION

▶ Recognition is the most important part of prevention. After identifying which foods, food additives, or specific environmental factors are involved, making modest changes often results in marked improvements, particularly in young children.

▶ Reduce the use of air fresheners, fabric softeners, and other sources of chemical vapors.

# FATIGUE

Fatigue refers to excessive tiredness that is out of proportion to a person's level of activity or exercise. In chronic fatigue syndrome (CFS), also known as myalgic encephalo-myelitis (ME), fatigue is usually not relieved by rest. It is worse in the morning, shows gradual improvement during the day, but gets worse after minimal exertion. Severe exertion can leave a patient bedridden for days.

**Causes** Fatigue is extremely common and is a symptom of many diseases. In one survey in the United States, 50 percent of patients admitted to a hospital gave fatigue as one of their major symptoms. Fatigue commonly accompanies hay fever and other allergic reactions caused by airborne allergens and such chemicals as formaldehyde. Hidden food allergy (particularly, but not only, to milk products) and environmental allergies are often associated with fatigue. Disturbed sleep and insomnia, resulting directly or indirectly from allergic reactions, can cause tiredness and lethargy.

Chronic fatigue syndrome is now recognized as a definite and very disabling illness, though it is still not fully understood. In the early stages it is important to rest. Later, muscles must be gently exercised, increasing the exercise gradually but being careful not to worsen symptoms. Patients with CFS who also have other symptoms are often helped by identifying and dealing with allergies.

**Treatment** There is no specific drug treatment for fatigue. Tranquilizers often make symptoms worse, but anti-depressants can be helpful, especially when depression is also a factor. Fatigue often disappears when the allergic causes are identified. Supplements of essential fatty acids, magnesium, and vitamin $B_{12}$ can be useful. Chinese energy tonics containing ginseng sometimes help. Herbs like passion flower and valerian are recommended to induce a good night's sleep. Acupressure may help boost energy levels.

*WHEN AND WHERE?*
*Think about foods and environments that seem to affect your fatigue. You might identify times when and places where it is worse; these could give you clues about the triggers that may be causing your problem.*

---

## PREVENTION

▶ Avoiding sweets is a good idea. Fatigue is sometimes associated with low blood sugar levels, which can follow a sugar boost. Have savory snacks, such as crackers, nuts, seeds, cheese, and popcorn, and unsweetened beverages between the main meals of the day.

▶ Keeping a food diary and then trying an elimination diet is often successful in reducing fatigue, because the condition is common in cases of allergy and intolerance. Milk products are high on the list of foods that can cause fatigue, but certain grains, tea, coffee, and other foods can also be triggers.

▶ Undertaking an environmental cleanup to reduce exposure to inhalant allergens and chemicals both at home and work is also a good measure (see pages 64–71). If you have experienced improvement in the condition during a vacation in a totally different locale, this could indicate that your problem has an environmental cause related to inhalants, such as pollens or chemical fumes.

---

## TENSION AND FATIGUE

Fatigue sufferers often find that their tiredness is accompanied by a constant state of tension, leaving them feeling simultaneously tense and exhausted. This combination of symptoms is found in both adults and children, and it can form part of the constellation of symptoms involved in hyperactivity (see page 136). Sufferers often exhibit "allergic shiners"—dark circles under their eyes—that can act as a key marker for allergic fatigue.

# MIGRAINE AND OTHER HEADACHES

Many terms are used to describe headaches—constant, throbbing, aching, stabbing. They can affect one or both sides of the head and may spread down into the neck and/or shoulders. Migraine is a complex of symptoms, with headache the major one. Other symptoms include disturbed vision, nausea, vomiting, and hypersensitivity to light, noise, and movement.

Migraine can last from a few hours to two or three days, and is often followed by fatigue and hypersensitivity to stimuli. It rarely occurs before puberty, but children who have recurrent unexplained abdominal pains may be predisposed to migraine.

**Causes** A headache can be a symptom of many different conditions, such as infections, stress, muscle spasm, and eye or ear problems, but most headaches are not accompanied by any demonstrable illness. Some

have environmental causes. Though the cause of migraines is not known, they are often provoked by environmental factors, including hormones, stress, and certain foods.

**Treatment** When treatable illnesses have been excluded as a cause, treatment usually concentrates on relieving symptoms using a non-steroidal anti-inflammatory drug or another painkiller. A variety of drugs may be used for migraine, including antinausea drugs and, in severe cases, strong analgesics by injection.

Yoga, t'ai chi, and the Alexander technique are all useful for relieving stress and helping prevent or relieve headaches. Feverfew is a well-established herbal remedy for migraine, and reflexology is often used to relieve pain and other symptoms. Many people have found osteopathy and acupuncture also beneficial in relieving headaches.

## PREVENTION

▶ The role of hidden food sensitivities in migraine has been established in trials involving both adults and children. In some cases simple changes may be sufficient, such as not skipping a meal or avoiding caffeine, cheese, or red wine. In other cases an elimination diet may be needed to identify the culprits that trigger migraine.

▶ If an elimination diet is needed, it may have to be undertaken with medical supervision because withdrawal reactions and the reactions to food challenges can sometimes be severe.

▶ Steps should also be taken to reduce exposure to chemicals and airborne allergens.

▶ Avoiding trigger foods can be just as effective with other sorts of headache as it is with migraine.

## A SIMPLE YOGA POSTURE FOR HEADACHE RELIEF

Yoga is an excellent therapy for sufferers of migraines and other headaches because it relieves muscular tension, often a cause of headaches. Shown below is a move

called a spinal twist with an added element, a pad between the shoulder blades—you can use a tightly folded sock—which customizes the pose for headache relief.

1 *Lie on your back with a folded sock or small pad positioned between your shoulder blades. Slowly bring your knees up and put your right arm behind your thighs, hugging your knees to your chest. Let your left arm lie at your side. Roll your head to the left, keeping your chin tucked in.*

2 *Move your left arm so that it is at right angles to your body. Exhale and, keeping your head turned to the left and your shoulders on the ground, roll your legs and hips to the right. Breathe in and out five times and then bring your arms and legs back to the center. Repeat to the opposite side.*

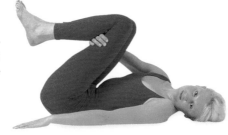

### HEADACHE AND MIGRAINE TRIGGERS

Alcohol, smoking, stress, and the contraceptive pill contribute to migraines and other headaches; food probably plays a part in at least 60 percent of cases. Chemicals and inhalant allergens can also be responsible. Foods recognized as triggers of migraine include coffee, chocolate, cheese, red wine, and citrus fruits, but any hidden food allergy can trigger the condition, as can sensitivity to pollens, house dust mites, animals, and volatile chemicals. Other types of headaches may result from tension, dental work, or physical problems that have caused the jaw or neck to become misaligned.

# Genitourinary Disorders

*Problems such as infertility and kidney disease fall outside the range of disorders normally attributed to allergies. However, in some cases, uncovering and avoiding allergic triggers can help to resolve apparently intractable conditions.*

## KIDNEY AND BLADDER PROBLEMS

Allergic reactions can lead to serious kidney problems, including fluid retention, blood or protein in the urine, and severe pain. Bladder symptoms—lower abdominal pain and difficulties with passing urine (the need is frequent, painful, and urgent)—may be caused by urinary infection, but the same symptoms can result from allergies. In children allergies can be a factor in bed-wetting, and in the elderly a worsening of stress incontinence. Kidney problems can be very serious and should always be reported to a doctor.

**Causes** The kidneys and bladder comprise the major excretory system of the body, which means that many allergenic substances pass through them. Bladder irritation may also be caused by toiletries applied around the genitals, fabrics used in underwear, and laundry detergents and fabric softeners. Foods, especially grains and fruits, are by far the most common cause of allergic bladder symptoms in children; medications may also cause problems.

**Treatment** One measure for relieving symptoms is to increase fluid intake to at least eight 8-ounce glasses a day. Liquids help wash the causes of

irritation away, whether they are bacteria or allergens. Another approach is to make your urine more alkaline by eating more alkaline foods, like vegetables, and reducing protein and cereal intake, or taking supplements of potassium or sodium citrate.

Homeopathic remedies like *Nux vomica* and *Apis mel* may help lessen the urge to urinate and relieve pain in the lower abdomen.

*HELP FOR URINARY PROBLEMS*
*Teas of couch grass, marsh mallow, parsley, or yarrow can soothe urinary problems but can also cause allergic reactions of their own; use them with caution.*

### PREVENTION

▶ Avoid strong soaps, detergents, and personal products. Wear cotton underpants, which can be washed at a very high temperature—at least 80°C (176°F)—to eliminate organisms such as *Candida*.

▶ Try to identify and avoid food triggers. This measure can make a dramatic difference with both bladder and kidney problems.

▶ For intractable bladder problems, treatment to prevent fungal overgrowth in the bowel may be needed.

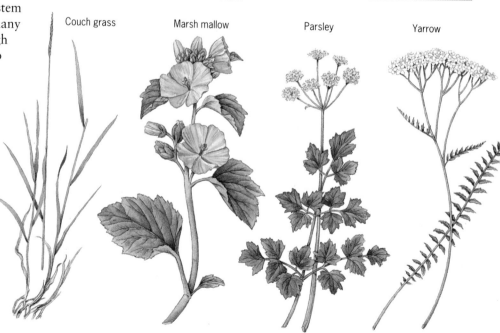

Couch grass    Marsh mallow    Parsley    Yarrow

152

# INFERTILITY

Infertility is defined as the inability of a couple to conceive after trying for at least a year, although the time interval is arbitrary. Some doctors insist on waiting longer before starting investigations, depending on the ages of the two people.

**Causes** The past 40 years have seen a significant reduction in sperm count in men. The reasons for this are not yet clearly established, but increased use of hormones, the effect of chemicals that mimic hormones, and exposure to pesticides are all suspected causes. A number of conditions can contribute to infertility in women, ranging from being underweight to infections that can block the fallopian tubes. Smoking, excessive drinking, and nutritional deficiencies damage the fertility of both sexes.

Allergy can play a part in some cases. Allergic infertility can be reversed if investigations identify sensitivities to foods, airborne allergens, or chemicals (or to a combination of them) and appropriate avoidance measures are taken. There was a case in which sensitivity to milk was shown to inhibit ovulation. In rare cases, a woman becomes allergic to her partner's semen, so the immune system attacks and destroys the sperm.

**Treatment** The first step usually is to eliminate infection and treat any other possible cause. If these measures are unsuccessful, hormonal therapy or various fertility treatments, such as artificial insemination or in vitro fertilization, may be tried. Taking supplements to rectify nutritional deficiencies and avoiding exposure to environmental allergens can be very successful in some patients. Acupuncture may also be helpful. Herbal remedies are generally not recommended.

*ALLERGY AND INFERTILITY*
*An allergist can help you identify foods or chemicals from your environment that might be causing or contributing to infertility. Avoiding them could be the best therapy.*

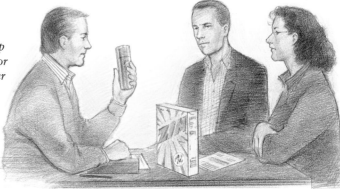

### PREVENTION

▶ Improving the diet and possibly taking supplements of vitamins, plus the minerals zinc, magnesium, and selenium—with the supervision of a doctor or dietitian; maintaining good general health and fitness; and not smoking are important for both men and women.

▶ Keeping the testicles cool by avoiding tight pants and hot baths can help men to keep up their sperm counts.

▶ Maintaining a healthy body weight and a balanced diet is essential for women looking to improve their fertility.

---

# VAGINAL INFLAMMATION

Vaginal inflammation (vaginitis) is characterized by soreness, itching, and discharge. It varies in severity from a slight nuisance to a debilitating handicap, with symptoms of cystitis and severe pain making sexual intercourse impossible.

**Causes** The most common cause is infection, particularly candidiasis, but vaginitis can also result from contact allergies to rubber; synthetic fibers, dyes, and finishes in fabrics; toiletries; and medications of any sort. Allergic reactions to contraceptives are becoming more common, particularly to the latex in diaphragms and condoms. Women can also become sensitized to their partner's seminal fluid. Foods, chemicals, and inhalants can all cause reactions in the vagina.

**Treatment** Infectious causes must be treated appropriately, but topical medication should be used with care because sensitivity to the product can easily occur. Yogurt with live cultures and a diet low in sugars and refined starch are effective natural treatments for candidiasis, but you should seek medical advice for any vaginal inflammation. An herbalist may advise soothing pessaries or douches to correct any imbalances in the vaginal secretions.

### PREVENTION

▶ Identifying and avoiding irritants and allergens is essential. Think about everything that comes into contact with your genitals, including clothes and the detergents in which they are washed.

▶ Consider hidden food allergies and inhalant allergens as well, especially if vaginitis is seasonal.

# Respiratory Disorders

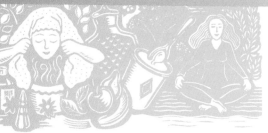

*This group includes some of the classic allergic disorders, such as hay fever and asthma. Disorders of the ears and sinuses also fall under this heading because they are areas related to the respiratory tract and involve irritation of mucous membranes.*

## HAY FEVER AND RHINITIS

Rhinitis symptoms typically involve the nose—itching, sneezing, runny and/or congested passages—and may be accompanied by eye symptoms, such as itching, sensitivity to bright light, and discharge. Hay fever is a seasonal allergic rhinitis, which often occurs during the spring or summer months, particularly the grass pollen season, but it can afflict someone throughout most of the year. With hay fever the palate and throat may also itch, and the patient may feel unwell, with headaches and fatigue.

**Causes** Hay fever during May and June is usually caused by exposure to grass pollen. At other times it can be due to tree or ragweed pollen or to seasonal mold spores. Perennial rhinitis, in which symptoms persist all year-round, is caused by one or more of the following: dust mites, pet hairs, mold spores, chemical fumes, and hidden food allergy.

**Treatment** Treatment with nasal decongestants and antihistamines is usually sufficient. Capsules of freeze-dried nettle leaves are a good alternative to antihistamines. Inhaling the steam from boiled water infused with 4 to 10 drops of peppermint oil helps relieve congestion. The homeopathic remedies *Gelsemium* and *Arsenicum album* are said to relieve blocked and runny noses, sore eyes, and sneezing. Regularly instilling a few drops of salt water (½ teaspoon per cup of warm water) in each nostril can also bring relief.

### PREVENTION

▶ Avoiding inhaled allergens will prevent symptoms in 50 percent of perennial rhinitis cases; detecting and avoiding trigger foods will help in most of the remaining cases.

▶ Milk is a leading trigger of rhinitis. Both environmental measures and an elimination diet are often needed, but of the two, detection and avoidance of trigger foods like milk are more likely to bring dramatic improvement.

▶ Desensitization (see page 48) is often effective, but takes time.

**FIRST LINE OF DEFENSE**
*Decongestants and antihistamines bring short-term relief for hay fever but have side effects.*

## SINUSITIS

If the mucous membranes lining the sinuses are inflamed, the openings can become blocked, causing a buildup of mucus. This may lead to pressure, pain, and possibly infection, or acute sinusitis.

**Causes** Sinusitis can be caused by bacterial infections of the membranes lining the sinuses, but allergic rhinitis is often to blame.

**Treatment** Antihistamines and decongestants bring short-term relief but they can exacerbate symptoms in the long run. Naturopaths recommend natural decongestants, such as fenugreek tea or inhaling steam, and natural antihistamines like vitamin C. These may be as effective as conventional medication, without the side effects. Sponging or splashing the face and sinus areas

### PREVENTION

▶ Most cases of sinusitis brought on by allergic rhinitis respond to the detection and avoidance of environmental triggers.

with water, alternating two minutes with hot water and one minute with cold, can provide relief. Antibiotics may be needed for acute sinusitis.

## ASTHMA

In people with asthma the airways in the lungs are hyperreactive and go into spasm, causing shortness of breath and wheezing as they become constricted and mucus is secreted. The condition is very common, and over the past 20 years its incidence has grown dramatically, especially among children—more than 5 million in North America alone now suffer with it.

**WARNING**

*Asthmatics should take great care when trying food challenges, even when they are investigating other conditions. A food challenge taken after avoiding a trigger for a week can cause unexpectedly severe reactions. Consult your doctor first.*

**Causes** The underlying cause of asthma is inflammation of the airways due to release of chemicals such as histamine. In the majority of asthmatics, release is provoked by reactions to one or more environmental allergens or foods, and by looking hard enough, the cause or causes can almost always be found.

**Treatment** Asthma is treated with a variety of drugs—primarily bronchodilators for quick relief and controller drugs, mostly corticosteroids, to prevent attacks. Nonsteroidal drugs, such as cromolyn sodium, may also be used. However, these medications are aimed at suppressing symptoms rather than attacking the causes of the problem. Drinking plenty of liquids, particularly hot liquids, can help clear mucus from the airways. Learning to relax your breathing is also a major step in reducing the severity of attacks.

**PREVENTION**

▶ Identifying and avoiding the triggers that cause asthma is the best prevention. The majority of asthmatics can be helped by taking basic steps to avoid the most common environmental triggers and the most common food allergens (see Chapters 3 and 4).

▶ Keeping fit and maintaining normal weight are other important factors in prevention. Fit people are better at extracting oxygen from the air they breathe, and slim people have less weight around the diaphragm, which makes it easier for them to breathe comfortably.

▶ Because magnesium deficiency makes asthma worse, a supplement of this mineral should be considered, as well as eating plenty of fresh fruits and vegetables.

## EAR PROBLEMS

Chronic infection of the middle ear, known as acute otitis media, is a common condition in young children but also occurs in adults. Inflammation of the inner ear is also a problem for adults and children, and can lead to permanent hearing loss.

**Causes** Ear infections can be caused by a virus or bacterium, usually one that has invaded the nose, throat, or sinuses first. However, the disorder can also result from an allergy, especially in children. Rhinitis, whatever the cause, leads to blocking of the eustachian tube and a buildup of fluid in the ear. Sometimes the fluid builds up to the point where the eardrum bursts.

**Treatment** Decongestants and antihistamines for mild cases. Homeopaths suggest *Pulsatilla* to improve drainage and *Ferrum phos.* for earache. Gargling with warm salt water when ear pain begins may bring some relief.

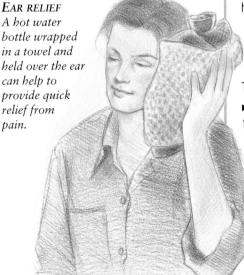

*EAR RELIEF*
*A hot water bottle wrapped in a towel and held over the ear can help to provide quick relief from pain.*

**PREVENTION**

▶ More than 80 percent of children with middle-ear infections have rhinitis, and when the causes of rhinitis are found and eliminated, hearing improves and infections diminish. In many instances airborne allergens are to blame, but in at least 10 percent of cases, the problem is due to Type B allergies to foods.

▶ Milk is often one trigger but other foods may also be involved. When milk products have to be avoided, they must be cut out completely. Children not drinking milk should probably take a calcium and magnesium supplement.

▶ It can help to eat more vegetables and reduce sugars and additives in the diet.

# GLOSSARY

**Allergen:** an *antigen* that causes an allergic reaction.

**Angioedema:** a reaction that causes swelling in the deeper layers of the skin, especially of the face and lips.

**Antibody:** a protein molecule made by the body in response to a foreign molecule, or antigen. Antibodies, which are programmed to recognize one specific antigen, belong to a class of proteins called *immunoglobulins*.

**Antigen:** any substance that elicits an immune response.

**Anaphylaxis:** a severe generalized allergic reaction that can lead to shock. If not treated, anaphylaxis can be fatal.

**Atopy:** a general tendency to overproduce *IgE*, and thus be highly allergic. Allergic reactions like hay fever are manifestations of atopy.

**Challenge:** exposing an allergy sufferer to a suspect substance—for example, a food or scent—in order to see if it provokes a reaction.

**Chronic:** a long-term and/or recurring health condition.

**Complement:** a group of chemical messengers in the blood that play a part in inflammation and the activation of *phagocytes* and other immune cells.

**Cytotoxicity:** the killing of a cell, whether by another cell, a cytotoxic T-cell, for instance, or a chemical.

**Dander:** tiny skin particles from animals, especially those with fur, that can cause an allergy in susceptible individuals.

**Dermatitis:** a general term for skin inflammation, including *eczema*. Some dermatitis results from an allergy, but often the cause is unknown.

**Desensitization:** a procedure, of which there are several different types, to reduce an individual's sensitivity to an allergen. Also called immunotherapy.

**Eczema:** a skin condition in which patches of skin become thickened, red, and itchy and that may erupt into blisters that weep and crust over.

**Edema:** swelling that results from fluid retention. It can be caused by kidney disease or by a food allergy or intolerance.

**Elimination diet:** a diet used to identify the foods responsible for delayed, or hidden, food allergies. People limit their diets to foods least likely to cause problems until symptoms diminish.

**Essential fatty acids (EFAs):** components of certain fats and oils that play an essential part in metabolic processes but cannot be made in the body. They are important for the health of cell walls, nerves, and some of the messengers in the immune system.

**Evening primrose oil:** oil from the seeds of the evening primrose. It contains the *essential fatty acid*, gamma-linolenic acid (GLA), helpful in relieving many allergy symptoms, including *eczema*.

**Food intolerance:** a term that can be used for all adverse reactions to foods not due to an obvious allergy, or just for those conditions that result from deficiencies in enzymes and interfere with digestion or metabolism of food.

**Gluten:** the main protein in wheat, also found in rye, barley, and some other grains to varying degrees; it must be avoided by sufferers of celiac disease.

**Hidden food allergy:** a reaction to a food in which the link between symptoms and ingesting the food is not clear. Symptoms may be vague, take a long time to develop, or affect parts of the body other than the gut.

**Histamine:** an important inflammatory chemical messenger. It is stored in granules in mast cells and released when they degranulate.

**IgE:** a type of *immunoglobulin* that is responsible for immediate allergy. IgE is usually carried on the surface of mast cells.

**Immune-mediated:** caused by specific reactions of cells or molecules of the immune system. Allergies, for instance, are immune-mediated.

**Immunoglobulin (Ig):** another name for the *antibody* class of proteins.

**Inflammation:** a response to injury, allergy, or infection in which the tissues of the body become painful, hot, red, and swollen. *Phagocytes* and other cells flow into the affected area to clean up and promote healing.

**Lymphocytes:** immune cells that react to foreign molecules, or antigens. They include B- and T-cells.

**Masked food allergy:** another name for *hidden food allergy*, in which the trigger is ingested frequently enough for the symptoms from one reaction to fade into the next set of symptoms.

**Phagocytes:** a group name for body cells that destroy foreign cells, particles, and molecules by engulfing and digesting them. Types of phagocytes include macrophages and polymorphs.

**Placebo:** an inactive treatment given in place of real treatment. In a double-blind trial, for instance, a subject may be given a sugar pill instead of a drug. When a placebo treatment provokes a change in symptoms, this is called a placebo effect.

**Polysymptomatic:** experiencing many apparently unrelated symptoms.

**Pseudoallergy:** when mast cells or other elements of the allergic response are triggered directly by a chemical and not by a normal allergic mechanism, the effects appear to be the same as an allergic reaction, but are said to be pseudoallergic.

**Radioallergosorbent test (RAST):** the name of a test used to detect levels of *IgE* antibody in a person's blood.

**Somatization:** the expression of psychological problems through physical symptoms. This term is used by some doctors to explain Type B allergy symptoms, which they argue have no physical cause.

**Tolerance induction:** the process whereby the immune system is encouraged to become tolerant of an *allergen*. Artificial tolerance induction is the aim of *desensitization*.

**Topical:** applied locally, rather than systemically, through inhalation, spraying, or rubbing in.

**Toxin:** a poisonous or harmful substance. Toxins may come from outside the body—from bacteria, wasp stings, plants, or chemicals, for example. They can also be produced by cells inside the body.

**Urticaria (nettle rash/hives):** a condition in which the skin becomes very itchy with swollen blotches known as wheals.

# INDEX

# ACKNOWLEDGMENTS

**Carroll & Brown Limited**
would like to thank
British Society for Allergy,
  Environmental and Nutritional
  Medicine, Southampton
Dr Sheldon Cohen, Scientific Advisor,
  National Institute of Allergy and
  Infectious Disease
Sharon Freed
Green and White Ltd
IDIS World Medicines
Margaret Moss
Sara Turner

**Editorial assistance**
Denise Alexander
Angela Newton
Laura Price

**Design assistance**
Mercedes Morgan
Karen Sawyer
Jonathan Wainwright

**DTP design**
Elisa Merino

**Photograph sources**
Cover K.H. Kjeldsen/Science Photo
  Library
  8  National Library of
     Medicine/Science Photo Library
  9  Kimishige Ishizaka, MD
 10  (Top) Wellcome Institute
     Library, London
     (Bottom) Frank Spooner/Hajdih
     Bruno
 16  Courtesy of the National
     Library of Medicine Collection,
     National Institutes of Health,
     Bethesda, Maryland, USA
 19  Eddy Gray/Science Photo
     Library
 25  B. Wittich/Custom Medical
     Stock Photo/Science Photo
     Library
 27  Telegraph Colour Library
 29  Dr Kari Lounatmaa/Science
     Photo Library
 30  Lori Adamski Peek/Tony
     Stone Images
 32  BSIP, LECA/Science
     Photo Library
 38  Reference material courtesy of
     Vega Grieshaber GmbH & Co
 34  Prof Gunnar Johansson
 37  Manfred Kage/Science
     Photo Library
 42  Carroll & Brown
 43  K.H. Kjeldsen/Science
     Photo Library
 51  James Strachan/Tony
     Stone Images
 54  David Stewart/Tony
     Stone Images
 56  Mary Evans Picture Library
 58  Eye of Science/Science
     Photo Library
 59  (Left) CNRI/Science
     Photo Library
     (Centre) Dr Jeremy Burgess/
     Science Photo Library
     (Right) David Scharf/
     Science Photo Library
 63  Images Colour Library
 68  Carroll & Brown
 72  CNRI/Science Photo Library
 74  Zigy Kaluzny/Tony
     Stone Images
 80  Chris Priest & Mark
     Clark/Science Photo Library
 81  Labat, Jerrigan/Science
     Photo Library
 84  Rex Features
 88  Andrew Syred/
     Microscopix Photolibrary
 93  Simon Fraser/Science Photo
     Library
 96  M. Ashley/Anthony Blake
 98  John G. Egan, Dublin/
     Hutchison Library
102  Eye of Science/Science
     Photo Library
103  Andrew Syred/
     Science Photo Library
104  Hutchison Library
112  Corbis-Bettman
114  Dr Jeremy Burgess/
     Science Photo Library
116  Wellcome Institute
     Library, London
120  (Top) Dale Durfee/Tony
     Stone Images
     (Bottom) Hutchison Library/
     Maurice Harvey
124  (Top) David Parker/Science
     Photo Library
125  Claude Nuridsany and Marie
     Perennou/Science Photo Library
126  The Movie Store
130  Ron Sutherland/Science
     Photo Library
132  Angela Hampton/Family
     Life Pictures

**Medical illustrators**
Paul Williams
Sandie Hill

**Illustrators**
John Geary
Nicola Gregory
Bill Piggins
Pond and Giles
Josephine Sumner
Anthea Whitworth

**Computer generated artwork**
Mick Gillah
Mirashade Ltd

**Photographic assistants**
M-A Hugo
Mark Langridge
Alex Franklin

**Hair and make-up**
Kim Menzies
Jessamina Owens

**Picture research**
Sandra Schneider

**Research**
Denise Alexander
Steven Chong

**Index**
Nadia Silver

75-009-3